"A fascinating, joyful social and personal history of an underrated drug. Zmith manages to capture not just the intriguing story of poppers and their role in queer life, but also something of their ineffable chemical pleasure."

— **HUW LEMMEY**, AUTHOR OF *UNKNOWN LANGUAGE*

"A pharmacornucopia of sensory pleasures, Adam Zmith's *Deep Sniff* is an entire queer curriculum opened up by poppers: an anti-skool of body chemistry, dance floor history, sci-fi physics, self-pleasuring craft design technologies, gymnastic artistry (courtesy of Luis Amália), and a queer literature of mutable masculinities. Celebrating the open, the voracious, and the capacious aspects of the QUILTBAG community and continuity, Zmith says RELAX!, linking the beautiful apertures of sphincters and wormholes into a cosmic as well as anti-capitalist, queer vision of possibility."

— **SO MAYER**, AUTHOR OF
A NAZI WORD FOR A NAZI THING

"Absorbing, riotous, keenly-researched and utterly celebratory, *Deep Sniff* is exactly the kind of queer history we need right now! Through the heady prism of poppers, Zmith explores the queer body with such curiosity and nuance – and explodes just how very political and ongoing the search for autonomous pleasure really is. *Deep Sniff*, with all its joyful openness and rigorous scholarship, brings what has existed in the margins for too long into the centre of the page with a dizzying and multifarious roar!"

— **RICHARD SCOTT**, AUTHOR OF *SOHO*

"A fascinating book!"

—**DAN SAVAGE**, AUTHOR OF *SAVAGE LOVE*
AND

"Adam Zmith's *Deep Sniff* is a fascinating dive into the history of a common, yet rarely remarked upon part of gay male life in the late twentieth and early twenty-first century: poppers. Deftly intermingling history, personal experience, and cultural commentary, *Deep Sniff* is a remarkable addition to queer history."
— **HUGH RYAN**, AUTHOR OF *WHEN BROOKLYN WAS QUEER*

"A beautiful exploration of a hieroglyph of marginalised pleasure. *Deep Sniff* is both a personal and cultural history of influence, and a shimmering investigation into the chemical facets of queer sociality. A must-read!"
— **PETER SCALPELLO**, AUTHOR OF *LIMBIC*

"What emerges on the pages of *Deep Sniff* is more than a dry historical survey. It's a riotous, unflinching defence of hedonism."
—**THE FACE**

"Brilliant. It's such a beautifully written journey through the history of poppers. I feel nostalgic, which a litany of past headaches tells me is effing misplaced. Highly recommended read."
—**JUNO ROCHE**, AUTHOR OF *QUEER SEX*

"The precise connection between poppers and potential queer liberation may seem fuzzy, but Zmith guides you by the hand each step of the way... The author is consistent in refuting the myriad limitations of identity, advocating a fluidity and nuance in gender and sexuality that's proving increasingly rare to find."
—**HUCK**

DEEP SNIFF

DEEP SNIFF

A HISTORY OF
POPPERS AND
QUEER FUTURES

Adam Zmith

Published by Repeater Books

An imprint of Watkins Media Ltd

Unit 11 Shepperton House

89-93 Shepperton Road

London

N1 3DF

United Kingdom

www.repeaterbooks.com

A Repeater Books paperback original 2021

2

Distributed in the United States by Random House, Inc., New York.

Copyright © Adam Zmith 2021

Adam Zmith asserts the moral right to be identified as the author of this work.

Also published in Spanish by Dos Bigotes, translated by Joan Daròs.

ISBN: 9781913462420

Ebook ISBN: 9781913462604

Printed and bound in the UK by TJ Books

CONTENTS

1. Undesirable Purposes

A woman wearing smart clothes is reading about the exhibition when she notices the creature. She steps back and watches carefully. The looming figure has pale skin and black body hair, and it wears a red leotard that is adorned with glistening rhinestones. It could be a normal guy with a beard in east London. But tonight in the gallery he is a hairy gymnast performing a routine among strangers.

A person in round specs pauses their conversation to watch the performer dip onto his hands and knees, press his belly to the floor, stretch his feet then his hands... mimicking the length of the line. It is a thin white strip, pasted onto the floor, and it measures 16.97056274847714 metres – slicing right through the gallery space. A pair of people drinking wine from paper cups try to ignore the performance, but they also realise that they are standing on the performer's line, and he is moving towards them. The creature-gymnast seems to balance, to fit all its twists and turns, its pointed toes and bent knees, onto that line.

The routine is that of a gymnast, yes, but also that of a dancer, of an actress on a stage, a person trying to live, a soul desperate to hit its marks on the line. The length is the same as the diagonal across the 12 x 12m square sprung floor where a gymnast usually shows her best skills. The line is a constraint on her power but also a channel for it. The creature brings all this meaning into the gallery tonight, at the opening of a group show that mostly comprises pictures and objects. As the visitors talk to each other the artworks are a backdrop – except for the gymnast who penetrates them in sparkling sweaty lycra. Concentrated, poised, mischievous, the performer is Luis Amália and he is showing us a life on the balance beam.

Amália conceived of this piece as part of his ongoing performance work that takes on various forms. His project is to express an embodiment of female gymnasts and actresses. What he feels for them is more than an affinity or an admiration. His work is not satire, not drag. When his obsessions coalesce into these precise, rehearsed manoeuvres across a film set or a gymnastics arena, they are moving as Amália feels. Never good enough. Desperate to connect. Waiting to be judged. And yet! His act of *performing* these moves on his line somehow eliminates the negative feelings; he is freed of them, for a moment.

If there is something queer here, it is an attitude. When we watch Luis, we are all moving with him, along the line, cutting through official space.

Looking into the history of poppers requires the same attitude, and that is why this book opens with Amália's performance of a piece he named *16.97056274847714*, which was performed in London at the Queer Art(ists) Now

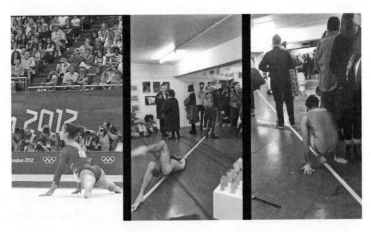

group art show in March 2020.[1] A history of poppers finds dozens of characters like Amália: different, daring, difficult. Whenever Amália performs, there is something "wrong" about him. His non-binary body is hairy, pale, perceived as male – and yet his soul is textured differently, light and dark, every gender and none. The creature is mesmerising: a utopia of being, free from categories, cutting through the expectations placed on him.

I wish I had seen Amália's performance when I was an adolescent, although I probably would have rejected it. As I grew up, I allowed categories and expectations far too much power, and I didn't have the courage of Amália to explore them artistically or to try to shake them off. I would have seen the freedom he implied, and turned away with teenage worry.

Growing up I panicked about who I desired, and I felt the pressure to be a "man", whatever that meant. It was bizarre to see that the men's bodies I wanted as my own were also the ones I wanted to touch. I knew that this meant other people would place me in a certain category, which bothered me. People see me as "gay" and as a "man". These categories were created long before I was. I inherited them, and had to fit them even though I didn't want to. Today, I'm never comfortable with them, but at least I have "queer", which is better. In this book I want to sniff out the multitudes contained in that word, and how this could help us to feel our way towards a future of uninhibited bodies and potential. To do that, I have to know where the idea of these labels "gay" and "man" came from in order to interrogate them. A history of poppers has some answers.

For a few years until 1976, the year my parents got married, the place to get poppers in London was Roland Chemist on Praed Street. This area, named Paddington after the railway station, was a busy district filled with shops, double-decker red buses, Ford Cortinas and Austin

Allegros. Billboards advertised mass products like Guinness and Levi's jeans. I can get a glimpse into poppers use at the time if I peer through the window of one small pharmacy in this bustling district. Roland Chemist, like any pharmacy in the UK, could lawfully sell amyl nitrite. The product was made by Burroughs Wellcome and marketed to those with heart problems. Amyl nitrite was sold in sealed glass ampoules, which were crushed by users to release the vapour of the liquid inside. This action made a "pop". This is how amyl nitrite, and similar substances, were packaged and used before the little brown bottles with safety caps came along. It's also how they got their name "poppers".

At the same time as Roland Chemist was known for selling amyl, the Boots Chemists in Piccadilly stocked twenty-four ampoules of amyl nitrite, which would last from four to six weeks. That's sales of around 250 per year.[2] The amount of amyl nitrite sold through Roland Chemist in Paddington was extraordinary. In one twelve-month period between 1975 and 1976, at the height of the pharmacy's poppers business, it sold 185,700 ampoules of amyl nitrite.[3] Let there be a gold plaque to Peter Beaton Lucas and Paul Roland Fletcher, the directors of the business, for their contribution to the enhancement of pleasure. Fletcher and Lucas also had two other shops on Earl's Court Road, close to a cluster of gay pubs including the Coleherne, which was popular with certain categories of gays including leathermen. They supplied their other shops through the Roland Chemist shop in Paddington.

Gay men would have made up the bulk of their customers. The pharmacists and shop directors were doing nothing wrong in selling amyl nitrite to anyone who asked: no law or regulation required a prescription for it. One of the pharmacists later said that he "did not ask questions" when asked for amyl nitrite, and usually just "sized people up and if they looked OK" he would make the sale.[4] But they knew who their customers were: a sales assistant at one of the shops later remarked that amyl nitrite was frequently sold to gay people. A box of a dozen ampoules cost no more than 65p to manufacture, and was sold at £1.10.

Lucas and Fletcher tread along the same line as Amália in his performance work. No one told them they couldn't do what they were doing. But their actions unsettled those around them, especially those with power. The problem started in 1975 when two men visiting Brighton walked into a pharmacy and asked for amyl nitrite. The pharmacist there asked for a prescription, so they told him they usually picked it up without one at Roland Chemist on Praed Street in London. Nice one, guys. This triggered a report to the police and an investigation by the Pharmaceutical Society, an industry body. The staff at Roland were spooked. They began to ask customers who requested amyl nitrite if they had a prescription. This must have troubled the gay men who were regular users. On December 29th, 1975, a volunteer at Gay Switchboard, the helpline, brought the problem to the attention of their comrades. He raised it in the pages

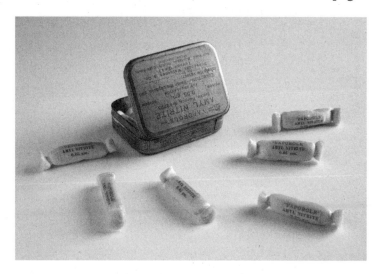

of the log book that they used to communicate with each other between shifts. The volunteer asked: "Where can you get Amyl Nitrate [sic] NOT on prescription since Roland Chemist requires one now[?]"[5]

Within six months, the supremely well-informed Switchboard volunteers had heard what was going on. One of them wrote in the log book on June 7th 1976:

> For those people who like "Poppers" and have had difficulty buying it at Chemists the reason is because the Chemists have received a letter, I think, from the National Health [Service], telling them of its misuse and asking them to use their discretion in serving people with it. It is apparently going to be added to the dangerous drug list soon.[6]

The heat was on. In September 1976, a committee at the Pharmaceutical Society considered Fletcher and Lucas's business. The committee concluded that in selling vast quantities of amyl nitrite, Fletcher and Lucas turned a blind eye to the improper use of the product. The two men were kicked off the pharmacists' register.

It took two years, but Fletcher and Lucas managed to overturn the verdict. The judges in the High Court did not rule that poppers were wonderful and safe and should be easily available. Instead, they upheld Fletcher and Lucas's appeal on the grounds that the members of the Pharmaceutical Society committee had done something unfair when considering the earlier case. To help them understand amyl nitrite, the committee members had consulted an edition of William Martindale's *Extra Pharmacopoeia of Unofficial Drug and Chemical and Pharmaceutical Preparations* – but they chose not to say so. This giant book, first published in 1883, synthesised all the recent advances in therapeutics.[7] It was an alphabetical catalogue of drugs, each listed with reference to published evidence and guidance on how to administer it. In *Martindale*, amyl nitrite was listed as a very safe drug that could be used against various problems including angina, but could be detrimental to health if used improperly.[8]

It was not the first time the British establishment had worried about amyl nitrite. In 1956, the Home Secretary, Gwilym Lloyd George, heard that "some chemists in the West End of London have been selling amyl nitrite in circumstances which suggest that it is not required for legitimate medical purposes".[9] He held off from taking action against this, though. Lloyd George agreed with the Poisons Board that in principle it was not right to use prescriptions to control substances that are not highly poisonous "simply because they are liable to be used for undesirable purposes". This might be the first free pass for poppers in history. (He was not so lenient with Ruth Ellis, a murderer, whose death sentence he refused to commute in 1955.)

But someone, somewhere, always wants to see sex as improper. Twenty years after Lloyd George's liberal approach, the members of the Pharmaceutical Society's committee assessing Fletcher and Lucas's case decided that sniffing amyl during sex was not a correct use of the stuff, so someone who did this could be harmed. In inferring what they wanted from *Martindale* without admitting it as evidence, the committee had made their own improper use of the book. This left Fletcher and Lucas with no way of debating the committee's claims. If they'd had that chance, they might have argued that by "improper use" the editors of *Martindale* meant drinking or eye drops. This is why the High Court upheld the pharmacists' appeal in the summer of 1978.

By this time in the USA, the business of poppers was much more aggressive. Whereas Roland Chemist salespeople knew their customers were gay men, they didn't market their product at them. In the USA, however, companies had begun to manufacture, distribute and advertise poppers as a product specifically for this demographic. Some of the famous brands from this time, Rush and Locker Room, endure to this day under the banner of a company called the Pacific Western Distributing Corporation (PWD), founded in 1976. It was the same year that other durable US brands were founded: Microsoft, Apple, Starbucks... To grow these businesses required obsessive minds focused on both product and experience, including the marketing of the product itself. For poppers, this is a credit that can go to a man called W. Jay Freezer. Within a year of founding PWD, he was claiming in the *Wall Street Journal* that his Rush brand of poppers ought to be sold alongside shampoo and macaroni cheese. "If Safeway supermarket customers want the product, I don't see why it couldn't eventually be sold there," he is quoted as saying in an article from October 10th, 1977.[10]

Freezer pioneered the advertising of poppers in gay newspapers and magazines, such as *Drummer*. Based in Los Angeles, this publication was aimed at leathermen and, according to Jack Fritscher, who became its editor-in-chief in 1977, it was started by John Embry simply as a way to promote his own business selling poppers and leather wristbands by mail.[11] The idea was to wrap reports and editorial columns on the leather scene around ads for gay products – and it worked. "Poppers kept *Drummer* flying high," wrote Fritscher in his history of the magazine, *Gay Pioneers*.[12] "Popper dealers paid a huge chunk of advertising dollars buying full-page display ads including expensive inside covers and back covers."

With Rush poppers, Freezer was among the biggest advertisers of *Drummer* and other gay magazines. Business boomed. Any number of ampoules Fletcher and Lucas sold in the UK through their pharmacy pales in comparison to what was happening in the USA, where poppers were already sold in branded bottles of 10-15ml, like Rush. One report put the figure for 1977 at four million bottles sold.[13] When Freezer spoke to the *Journal* that year, he claimed more than 60% of the market. This may be bluster, but it is also credible. Sniffing poppers in the 1970s was a huge part of gay life thanks to the ease of sending such a small product through the mail and the concentration of consumers in New York, Los Angeles and San Francisco. In New York, Pete Fisher, an activist and writer, was going to sex clubs where "poppers perfumed the thick, murky air".[14] This quote is taken from Fisher's 1980 novel *Dreamlovers*, which is based on his relationship with his lover Marc Rubin, another gay activist.

So poppers vapour filled the air over America and, as in the UK, authorities grew jumpy. The State of Connecticut banned the sale of poppers, based on assumed harm due to misuse – the same reason why the pharmacists were struck off in London. As an entrepreneur, Freezer was determined. A big part of his strategy was to sell poppers as a "room odouriser", not as an inhalant. And as well as aggressive advertising with erotic imagery and bizarre claims about enhanced masculinity, he did cheeky things like creating a new company and calling it Pharmex Ltd. This had the benefit of sounding like a more legitimate medical company and being a step removed from his distribution outfit. Through Pharmex, Freezer hired a bunch of experts to produce a report concluding that poppers were safe, and then he quoted from it when he spoke to journalists.

The report was authored by a group led by Mark Nickerson, a professor in the pharmacology department at McGill University in Montréal.[15] Nickerson's report seems initially very scientific and fair-minded in assessing the substance of amyl nitrite and its uses. But there is no mention in the body of the report about its sponsors

Pharmex and Freezer's poppers business, except a special thanks to PWD for assisting the study by supplying confidential information about its products. This omission may account for the fact that many of Nickerson's claims about the harmlessness of inhaling amyl nitrite in fact come from research on workers in a bottling plant. The subjects only inhaled amyl nitrite vapour in their ambient environment. The research on them was disingenuous because it assumed that poppers were indeed used as sold, that is as a "room odouriser".

But this is quite different to how users typically inhale, which is to hold a bottle of the liquid under one nostril, pressing closed the other, and taking a deep sniff of the rising vapour. The Nickerson report concludes that "it is difficult to envision any product with a better record of public safety". Freezer must have loved it – a report that exonerated his product by scientists who were supported by an apparently benevolent and medical-sounding company called Pharmex. He cited the report in an interview with Jane See White, a journalist from the Associated Press, for a story that made it into the Palm Springs *Desert Sun* newspaper on September 17th, 1979.[16] The peg for White's story was the death of a thirty-year-old man who died after drinking isobutyl nitrite, another substance with the same effect as amyl nitrite. Freezer advises against drinking "the disco drug", as the story calls it, saying that the Pharmex study found the only drawback from inhaling could be a headache. White's story did not state that Freezer had commissioned the study.

Freezer's business practices are emblematic of the early poppers industry. It all flew under the radar of most people, and even users of Rush were probably not minded to think too much about where their hit came from. However, a gay activist named Hank Wilson was on the case, self-publishing pamphlets against poppers and Freezer. The two squared off in an article in a gay newspaper in San Francisco called the *Sentinel*, published in 1981.[17] Wilson and Freezer wrote short pieces for and against poppers, and the Nickerson team even had a space too. (Again, no connection between Freezer and the Nickerson report was made.) When gay men began to die in the early 1980s in a way that was quickly related to sex, Wilson worked even harder, publishing more and more work linking deaths to poppers. Even to this day it is possible to find Wilson's work cited on websites that deny that the human immunodeficiency virus (HIV) causes the illnesses grouped as AIDS (more in Chapter 4).

Freezer died on March 27th, 1985, from an AIDS-related illness, aged forty-five.[18] While he had been a bombastic businessman, the entrepreneur who grew a bigger empire out of poppers had a milder persona. Joseph Miller began to manufacture poppers in the 1970s. Through the 1980s and 1990s, he became a rich and powerful figure in the business community in Indianapolis, where he based his company, Great Lakes Products. The company absorbed Freezer's after he died, and Miller even registered Freezer's old company name Pharmex in the state of Indiana.

Miller knew and funded local Democratic politicians. If you search for it, you can find a photograph of him with Bill Clinton, the US president. He gave money to the Damien Center, which was founded in 1987 to care for people living with HIV and AIDS-related conditions in Indianapolis. Today it serves more than four thousand people, many of them through its Joseph F. Miller Testing Center. You might wonder if the board members, or even Clinton, knew how Miller made his money. Well, plenty of people did ask questions; Miller was frequently the subject of investigation and rumour. In the 1970s there was a paedophile case, later dropped, naming him as a person of interest. By the time of his suicide in 2010, he was a deeply controversial figure in Indianapolis. Blog posts reporting on his death, and the comments beneath them, range from tributes to his warmth, generosity and thoughtfulness to allegations of paedophilia and the manic statement "JOE MILLER WAS ONE OF THE GREATEST MEN WHO EVER LIVED".

The strongest rumour about Miller, reported in the local press, was that he died at a time when his business was under investigation by federal authorities, according to his friends who knew that some of his premises had been raided. In fact, Miller's death and the rumours alone were enough to impede the supply of poppers into the market in 2010. Miller's business, it seemed, teetered on the balance beam. For a few months after he died in August 2010, poppers users found it hard to get hold of Rush, Freezer's brand that Miller's company was by now making, along with Quicksilver and Hard Ware. Sellers, online and those with shops, removed what products they did have from sale, and shortages were reported and discussed online in forums. Miller had already been fined by the US Consumer Product Safety Commission in 1994 for exporting poppers,[19] and now, it seemed, his business was threatened again. Who knew who might be next: sellers? Users?

It is hard to know whether sellers acted alone in pulling Miller's products, or whether his company also struggled to supply them immediately after his death. In any case, sellers were cautious for a while. By the end of 2010 supply was back to normal. The website for Rush, which links to authorised sellers, is still titled "PWD BRANDS ARE BACK" as of 2021, with PWD standing in for Pac-West Distributing, the company originally set up by Freezer.

The purpose of this short history of the industry and the people behind it is to reveal something of the relationship between commerce, regulation, and pleasure. The big story of business in the twentieth century is how capitalists and product developers created group identities they could market to, from housewives to teenagers, from Guinness drinkers to Ford drivers. Entrepreneurs like Freezer and Miller did the same thing for gay men, with poppers. It may have started as a Victorian medicine (Chapter 2), but it morphed into a feature of a sexual sub-culture and, for some, an identity (Chapter 3).

That brief business history also hints at one of the most distinctive features of poppers: the way that their own identity, their use, their category, exists outside of the law. The small brown bottles with jazzy labels are available over the counter in sex shops and convenience stores in the UK and USA. But this is only thanks to a pact between authorities and sellers. Everyone agrees to say that these products are not for human consumption, which means they are labelled with fake uses like "room odouriser" and "boot cleaner". In this way, the products are lawfully sold, bought and possessed. The authorities turn a blind eye to the fact that every single bottle contains a vapour that is sniffed by humans... except for the ones that are bought by mistake. They may be the only product that the state allows to be sold on a lie. Perhaps Lloyd George started this open secret from his office in Whitehall when he looked the other way after learning that people were buying amyl nitrite for an "undesirable purpose".

You might say that poppers fumes became incorporated into the body of the gay community; their ubiquity influenced even those who didn't use them. Like medicines, cosmetics, hormones, processed food, poppers penetrated a people. At the very least, the magazine ads that showed poppers users as muscly men with motorbikes entered readers' minds – and wielded a kind of biopolitical power, influencing how some of us think of ourselves, as sexual objects and as men (more in Chapter 3). Like Tom of Finland's drawings, these ads portrayed men who had dinner-plate pecs, leather chaps, and a desire to be fucked. It may seem like a subversive combination, but it created a standard for gay men that was almost as limiting as the standard of being strong and straight. "The biomolecular and organic structure of the body is the last hiding place of these biopolitical systems of control," writes Paul B. Preciado in his book *Testo Junkie*. "This moment contains all the horror and exaltation of the body's political potential."[20]

Let Preciado's claim that this is both a horror and an exaltation echo through these pages. Like any drug, poppers are a good thing and a bad thing. Or perhaps neither of these things, except when thinking makes it so. The project in this book is not to make a case for or against poppers. My desire is to think through that binary, and others. As the following chapters will show, poppers vapour is present in our lives, like it or not, usually as just a bit of fun. Few people think twice about poppers. Most people don't even know they exist, but many are using them. The annual report from the UK Home Office on drugs misuse found in 2016 that one in twelve people had used amyl nitrite.[21] (The Home Office stopped asking about amyl nitrite on subsequent reports.)

The little brown bottles are among us. You might know about poppers because Chantelle from down the road brought them to the corner of the school field and you all sniffed and felt weird and funny and that was that. Or because you worked in a queer bar and poppers helped you to bond with colleagues. Or because you need to sniff them tonight in order to relax your bumhole so you can be penetrated there. You might sniff them when you're dancing in a nightclub. This use has gone in and out of fashion for decades now. You might have done that in the late 1990s, when Ecstasy fell away. You could have been huffing the stuff in a sex club in the 1970s in San Francisco, and never imagined that the craze for poppers would have lasted this long or indeed that there would be a book about them. You might have poured a bottle of them into a big glass of Coca-Cola, shook it up for the fizz, and inhaled the sweet popping vapour for an extra kick. Or maybe you like to drip the stuff onto a sock which you roll up and place in your mouth. You might do that especially if you have a kink for feet, and you use someone else's sock after they've worn it for a few days... Humans and their objects are versatile. You might swallow the liquid, but then you'd be dead.

You might be a woman or a non-binary person, an intersex or transgender person, queer or asexual, straight, polyamorous, monogamous... or you just might be open to sniffing your feelings to convey you into a future regardless of descriptions and categories. Perhaps what you have is a private pattern, a way of keeping your little bottle concealed in the back of the fridge. You might take it out a few hours before you plan to use, building up your anticipation of a night spent blissfully alone, huffing and wanking. Or maybe you'll meet others online doing the same, watching them through the black mirror.

Pubs exist for drinking alcohol, clubs for dancing, petrol stations for refuelling. The only time poppers are the centre of an activity is in online video rooms that are shared among serious users (Chapter 7). Most of the time, poppers are peripheral. Even in a sex shop in a country where it is possible to sell them, they are discreet: small bottles usually held behind plastic or an assistant. The brands try hard to shout at the potential buyer with names like FIST, BRAIN FUCK and BANG!!. They use garish or extreme imagery. But their graphic designers are limited to such a tiny label, which has little power in a shop filled with outsized dildos and rubber body suits. These miniature artworks cut through the official space of the shop with labels that lie. Sellers rely on the fact that everyone who needs to know, knows.

Poppers are a giggle, but also a significant occupant of many lives, by the bedside and in the internet shopping history. It is surprising that a vapour from a tiny bottle can become a part of a people, but I hope these chapters will show you how. They are not love letters to poppers, or warnings for that matter; they are just facts and thoughts, assembled. This book began as a talk I gave in the basement of the Rose Lipman Building in Dalston as part of the Fringe! Queer Film & Arts Festival in 2019. The building was originally built as a library, but I used its space to tell a story that was not yet a book. Six months later, Amália would stick his white line to the floor in the same space as it was transformed into an art gallery for the Queer Art(ists) Now show. Amália's addition was to use the building as a gymnastics arena and a stage. The venue is not the only thing that links Amália's piece of work and this one. In fact, it was a sprout from a one-hour show that he and I had written together, called *Stigma*. We were also partners, and knowing his body and his soul got me thinking. I opened this chapter with his performance of *16.97056274847714* because it was an apparition of what would become the theme of this book.

I set upon a history of poppers because I wanted to know more about where poppers came from, how they shifted from angina relief to "poppers", and to document their place in our culture. Poppers are used by all sorts of people. So this story is about people who are queer, undecided, intersex, lesbian, transgender, bisexual, asexual and/or gay – that is, those of us who find community in the QUILTBAG, plus other humans and even aliens. But poppers are most heavily associated with gay men in rich countries in the West such as the UK and USA, thanks to entrepreneurs like Miller and Freezer. These labels are all part of my story too, which is why I focus on them in this book. So my gaze is on the gay men. If I want to cause trouble to our labels, I have to start with the ones that I use for myself. Being a gay man is my lineage, and artists like Amália inspire me to bend the line I'm supposed to be on. If I can stand in that gallery space, as I did, and watch Amália's free queer soul made manifest, I want to be able to do the same for mine. I want to use the way that poppers free me for forty-five seconds from these ideas that I am "gay" or a "man". Amália can find a queer human soul trapped inside the body of a gymnast who grins even as she lands with a toe out of line; I want to find the same in many more of us.

I may have been someone who has used his body for an undesirable purpose. If you say so. It is the project of this book to think about the purpose of our bodies, how we use them, and how we pose on Amália's line. The establishment has maligned the undesirable purposes of queer people, or excluded them. That is why so many of us feel like the "scarred bodies" hanging in the "popper-fog" described by Richard Scott in his epic poem of gay life, "Oh my Soho":

> ... I'm chock-full of shame, riven with dark man-
> jostling alleyways, a treasure map of buried trauma. In you
> I have spent my life – drunk, poppered up, tarnished,
> tear-stained,
> corroded, Eros
> -like.[22]

I do not see Scott's persona as corroded when he steps through history in this brilliant poem. I see him as full of potential, full of his own biopolitical power. His body is poppered-up, and present for nothing but connection. Let that be a theme of these chapters, too. Pleasure after pleasure through improbable connections. I would like to give your mind the experience that many bodies have when they are poppered-up: full of potential, seeking connection, and with the idea of the self falling away. All the best drugs give us this experience, of course, just as all the best performers do – like Amália, stepping along his line in a leotard, troubling the people in the gallery. Refusing categorisation, as our bodies do on their freest days, Amália performed a moment of queer potential. Entrepreneurs may have commercialised this by packaging hits of freedom and momentary utopia into small bottles, but the potential was there in our bodies all along.

After a busy opening night, Amália was due to repeat the same routine during the group exhibition, every day at 16:00:97, revealing his queer soul sixteen times for sixteen minutes. But it was March 2020, and London had begun to try to curb a virus. He turned up at the right time for the next few days, desperate to connect, with fewer and fewer viewers each day, and then the exhibition closed early. London locked down. Amália's queer utopia vanished, and we scurried away to our private boxes. Alone in mine, I began to write these pages.

The singer prefers shadow. I can barely see his face. When there is light in the show, it flashes from behind him. I'm thirty metres away from the stage, bodies knocking against me, ready for a rush. I brought poppers with me because I first heard this music used illegally on a porn compilation. The maker of the video had overlaid the clips with text and timed instructions on when to sniff. Here come the same beats now, produced live. Stage smoke clots the air. In the darkness, the three musicians are making a sound named TR/ST.

The singer's slithering lyrics are about shame taking hold… and a promise of hope without shame. The music is clear, pure, unencumbered. The sound is a laser beam through the smoke. I stop trying to use my eyes, and I feel the swell of the people around me. One is Jose, whose body moves with mine. We are nudged by others, too, and by the sound made on the stage. Darkness and bliss.

The singer's weird falsetto is a comfort and a connection. He says he is mercy, he is muscle, and this is how he touches his audience. Jose and I sniff poppers. Our bodies press. Everything is irresistible. Jose's hands, then lips, then skin. Jose and I are groping each other as the rush suffuses our bodies. This is a momentary world, the few seconds of rush, the ninety minutes of the show; it will all dissipate and the air outside will cloud everything once again. For now, in this moment, it is a shameless world imagined by dark figures on a stage, born through smoke, a promise made real.

It feels like grabbing something from the future, grabbing a few seconds of who we want to be. We become our potential. No suffering, only pleasure. The sensation is so, so brief.

2. Two Body Innovators

Have you ever seen bromine? It is an angry liquid, the colour of congealed blood.

At room temperature you have to store it in a sealed container, such as a glass ampoule. This is how you stop it turning to vapour. Bromine is so volatile that if you pour the reddish-brown fluid, you will see orange fumes rising, spoiling for a fight. Bromine is a natural element seeking connection. It seems to be alive, and full of potential.

Bromine and poppers share a connection in a man called Antoine Jérôme Balard. In 1826, Balard found a substance in seawater near his hometown of Montpellier in France, and after some studies he realised that this substance was a new element, bromine. (It had been isolated in Germany around the same time by Carl Jacob Löwig, who shares the title of discoverer.) Balard was an eccentric scientist who lived in an unheated garret above his laboratory. He started as a small-town pharmacist and rose to the Sorbonne, the most prestigious academic institution in France.

A few years after finding bromine, Balard passed nitrogen fumes through amyl alcohol. The process produced a curious liquid that gave off a pungent vapour. Balard must have moved his nose over this vapour and inhaled – it made him blush. "Nothing else has ever done that to me," he told a colleague, according to Thomas Dormandy in his book *The Worst of Evils: The Fight Against Pain*.[1] "I am a shameless character. I don't blush easily."

The year was 1844. Balard guessed that inhaling the vapour had dilated his blood vessels and lowered his blood pressure. He could not imagine a use for it. That task would be taken up by someone else. Just as Balard shared daddy duties for bromine with Löwig, he would co-parent amyl nitrite too, but after a lag. As Balard was co-discovering amyl nitrite in 1844, a baby was born in Scotland and named Thomas Lauder Brunton. This baby would grow up to become a doctor and an experimentalist who built on Balard's earlier discovery.

Brunton is the first of two body innovators I'd like to think about here. I do not think it is too much to say that he handed us every poppers rush we feel today.

In 1866 Brunton was the kind of bright, impatient medical student who just wants to make people feel better. In Brunton's day therapies took too long to move from the lab to the bedside, and were too often applied by doctors who did not understand exactly how a therapy might work.

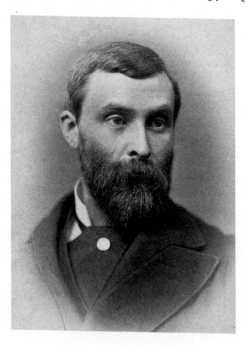

To Brunton, therapeutics was a poor science, and this bugged him while he walked the corridors of the Edinburgh Royal Infirmary during his medical training.

Take foxgloves, or *digitalis*. The plant had long been known as a folk remedy for people with heart problems. In 1785 the scientist William Withering published the first work on it as a medicine. And although doctors had used *digitalis* for some time before Brunton began his own training, the exact way it worked was not yet known. Nor was it being used systematically as a treatment. So Brunton took *digitalis* as the subject of his thesis, even testing it on himself. As well as seeking to understand how *digitalis* worked on the heart, he also used the project to take issue with the entire profession he was attempting to join. Brunton's thesis claimed that therapeutics was moving far slower than physiology and pathology, as seen in the example of *digitalis*. Doctors were just using trial and error in trying different drugs on different patients, he argued, without establishing standard therapeutic pathways.

"Turning from this unsatisfactory method," Brunton wrote, "we begin anxiously to look for one of a more rational character, which shall be based not only on a knowledge of the changes induced by disease, but on a minute and accurate acquaintance with the action of the remedies which we prescribe for its cure."

His audacity paid off. For his thesis, Brunton was awarded a gold medal from the university. It must have boosted the confidence of the young physician. The potential to convert discoveries into treatments that were founded in physiological understanding was immense. After *digitalis*, another substance was waiting to be exploited. In particular, Brunton was looking for something that would benefit patients who suffered with chest pain when not enough blood was flowing into their heart muscle. The problem was named as angina pectoris, but doctors did not have a reliable way of easing it. Angina patients were then sometimes treated by controlled bleeding, but it did not always work. Of his angina patients, Brunton wrote: "Few things are more distressing to a physician than to stand beside a suffering patient who is anxiously looking to him for that relief from pain which he feels himself utterly unable to afford."[2]

Brunton's distress brought him to amyl nitrite, first produced in the year of his own birth by Balard. There was still no known use for the smelly vapour beyond making chemists blush when they inhaled it. But Brunton had been reading the work of one such chemist, Benjamin Ward Richardson, who had spent some time observing its effects on rabbits and frogs, cats and dogs – and even his friends.

Not everyone who sniffed Richardson's amyl nitrite was a willing research subject. One friend saw a bottle of the stuff on Richardson's shelf while the scientist was out of the room briefly, and took a whiff. When Richardson returned, the friend was inhaling more and more deeply, and his face and neck had turned the colour of raw beef. Richardson tried to wrestle the bottle from him. The man, perhaps the world's first poppers pig, eventually gave it up, suddenly speechless, and needing support from a nearby table. "I shall never forget the gallop of that man's heart," wrote Richardson. "As he leaned against a table, the table vibrated and recorded visibly the pulsations." He led the friend out into the open air who, after a moment of depression and a loss of power (we've all been there), came around.

Richardson was perplexed. He sniffed it more than forty times himself – for science, I presume. He coaxed friends into joining him. And of course he did all sorts with animals. He began chucking rabbits into boxes pumped with amyl nitrite vapour and even injected the liquid into cats. Administering the stuff in various ways to his furry research subjects, he noticed "temporary excitement" that seemed to subside within minutes. Some of the animals died, especially when he made them drink it. And sometimes they came back to life. One frog that Richardson had left for dead after giving it amyl nitrite actually reanimated after nine days.

But it was the exact effects on blood vessels and muscles that Brunton took an interest in, as he read Richardson's work. Richardson documented one observation on a cat that had been trapped in a jar along with some amyl nitrite vapour. "Death took place within two minutes," he wrote – though quite how he was defining death is unknown. The animal's breathing had ceased, and the pupils had dilated, and Richardson and his colleague did not seem to wait long before opening up the poor creature's chest. "The heart was contracting vigorously," he wrote in his notes. Soon the breathing muscles began spontaneously to contract, moving the ribs and diaphragm. A muscle in the half-dead animal's thigh contracted too. These signs of life continued for an hour and twenty-four minutes.

So the blood vessels and muscles were clearly impacted by amyl nitrite, and they were the target that Brunton was looking for – a way to lower a patient's blood pressure without bleeding them. "As I believe the relief produced by the bleeding to be due to the diminution it occasioned in the arterial tension," he wrote, "it occurred to me that a substance which possesses the power of lessening it in such an eminent degree as nitrite of amyl would probably produce the same effect, and might be repeated as often as necessary without detriment to the patient's health."[3] This is why frogs are so important. The skin in their webbed feet is thin enough for you to see their capillaries. Perhaps frogs' feet would enable a scientist to observe the effect of amyl nitrite in the blood vessels of a living creature.

Brunton, the doctor who was looking for a way to ease blood flow to an angina patient's heart, read that

Richardson saw the capillaries in frogs' feet dilate when he gave them a sniff of amyl nitrite. "The rate of motion of blood is immensely quickened," Richardson wrote. This must have been what was happening in Richardson and his mates as they huffed too. He had noticed that a person's face became suffused with blood. When he gave it to a bald man, he saw the same effect practically over his whole head. Some humans reported feeling heat, others a tingling. "When these symptoms are at their height, a peculiar sensation is felt in the head, a sensation of tightness across the forehead, of fullness, giddiness, and prostration, but with no acute pain," wrote Richardson. These words gave Brunton his idea for a body innovation.

In reporting the effects of amyl nitrite, Victorian researchers made no mention of sexual arousal or the sudden need to be fucked. Despite observing "prostration" in some of his experimental human huffers, Richardson did not extend his studies to the effect on their bum muscles. He left behind a trail of cat corpses and energised bunnies, but no diagrams of beautiful puckering arseholes. Brunton never got into the bum game either, at least according to his notes. But in the winter of 1866, while a medical student in Edinburgh Royal Infirmary, he met a patient called William H. This young man was only twenty-six but already had trained as a blacksmith and then switched to toll-keeper. His first job may have required too much exertion for him to continue, because Brunton's notes reveal that William suffered from heart trouble.

When Brunton met him, William had recently been hit by a dull heavy pain about the left nipple, every three days or so, lasting for at least half an hour. The pain had come on after years of infrequent attacks ever since he'd suffered from rheumatism as a child. After a three-week hospital stay earlier in the spring, William was back just before Christmas. Doctors gave him aconite, which slows the heart rate, and *digitalis*. When neither worked, Brunton gave him brandy. The strong stuff didn't help either, so there was only one thing for it.

The experiment was not a stab in the dark. Brunton acted in a way that was consistent with his wishes to take basic research from the lab to the bedside, and only with a decent understanding of the actual effect in the body. He had read in Richardson's work that amyl nitrite dilated blood vessels and had even discussed the effect with his colleague in Edinburgh, Arthur Gamgee, who had made some unpublished measurements of this effect.

Brunton obtained some amyl nitrite from Gamgee, who made it for him, and consent for an experiment from his supervising physician. And this is how Brunton came to give his patient William amyl nitrite. On March 12th, 1867, Brunton observed:

> The pain came on as usual at 3am. A few drops of nitrite of amyl were put on a towel and inhaled by the patient. The primary effect noticed was a suffusion of the face, and the patient felt a glow over his face and chest. The pain disappeared almost simultaneously with the occurrence of these phenomena, but returned in three minutes. He then inhaled five drops more; the pain again disappeared and did not return.[4]

The relief did nothing to solve the underlying problem, but it certainly eased the pain. The doctor seemed to flipflop between making William sniff amyl nitrite and giving him a couple of fingers of brandy. But for sure, the amyl nitrite worked. Brunton wrote that the pain came on night after night, and always disappeared when William inhaled the vapour rising from a towel soaked in amyl nitrite. Within a month they had found a new method of inhalation – one that poppers pigs today might recognise. On April 10th,

Brunton observed, "Patient continues to have the pain every night, and instead of inhaling the nitrite of amyl from a cloth, does so from the bottle. Two or three inhalations usually suffice to relieve the pain."

The effect of amyl nitrite on Brunton's patient seemed magic. As a doctor, he must have felt the relief from his own suffering at witnessing a patient's difficulties. And as a scientist he must have felt gratified to see that applying the growing understanding of amyl nitrite could improve a patient's life. Brunton went straight to the *Lancet* with the news of having treated William. His paper, "On the use of nitrite of amyl in angina pectoris" was published in 1867.

There was nothing gay about amyl nitrite in 1867. In fact, there was little gay about Edinburgh, where Brunton lived and worked. Of course men there shagged each other, and women too, despite Queen Victoria's famous lack of imagination. But there is little trace of these private acts. Small numbers of prosecutions for sodomy between men are the only sign of what we now might think of as gay life. Indeed, it would be decades before something we could call gay life came to bloom in Scotland, and then more before the vapour sniffed by William would become a part of it.

And yet, Brunton shares the year of his discovery of amyl nitrite as an angina treatment with a leap forward in gay rights. Brunton's paper came out in 1867, the same year as the most important moment in the history of sexual freedom.

As Brunton submitted himself to his professional peers as having made a clinical breakthrough, another man in another country entirely stood up before his own peers. Karl Heinrich Ulrichs was a lawyer from the Kingdom of Hanover. Ulrichs thought that laws around public decency unfairly criminalised sex acts between men and were driven by prejudice. He was worried that if Prussia continued to expand, including into Hanover, it would also extend its outright ban on sodomy. Ulrichs took his arguments to a conference of the Association of Jurists, held in Munich in 1867. He stood before a room of five hundred jeering lawyers and made a declaration. In effect, he said: "I'm gay, and the law is an ass."

What links these remarkable triple-named men, Thomas Lauder Brunton and Karl Heinrich Ulrichs, is that in the same year they both saw the potential of our bodies to be eased from suffering and to live fuller lives. Brunton and Ulrichs were innovators who have especially helped queer souls to enjoy their bodies, individually and with others.

We have seen how Brunton's experimentalist approach found the first use for amyl nitrite. So now let us backtrack to look at how Ulrichs came to make his famous speech in 1867. Aged twenty-three, Brunton was at the start of a promising career. But Ulrichs' chosen career was already over, even though he was only forty-two.

Ulrichs was born into a family that was conservative, Christian and professional. It would have been expected of a young man like him to train as a bureaucrat or clergyman. So at nineteen he enrolled at the University of Göttingen. He studied law and came to favour the idea of a unified German-speaking state comprising the various kingdoms such as his own, Hanover. This set him against the expansionism of Prussia. Ulrichs got into this debate while at university, where he also discovered his desires:

I was at a dance but among the dancers there were about twelve young, well-developed and handsomely uniformed forestry pupils. Although at earlier dances no one caught my attention, I felt such a strong attraction that I was amazed... I would have flung myself at them. When I retired after the ball, I suffered true anxieties in my bedroom, alone and unseen, solely preoccupied by memories of those handsome young men.[5]

Ulrichs kept his eye on the prize, though: winning honours for his essays and good marks. After university, he found respectable work as a bureaucrat, and began to climb the ranks. By 1854 he was an assistant judge in the Hanoverian Ministry of Justice. But this was when he was forced to resign. "Ulrichs is said often to be seen in the company of lower-class persons under circumstances that allow one to conclude a close connection," read a report passed to his employers. "[T]here came to my attention a rumour that Ulrichs practices unnatural lust with other men."

Hanoverian law allowed the imprisonment of anyone found guilty of "unnatural lust under circumstances that cause public offense". Although Ulrichs was never committed of any crime, a police official confirmed the report – and this was enough to worry his bosses. Gossip that one of their number favoured unnatural lust could have brought the ministry into disrepute. His body was too dangerous; his position untenable.

Ulrichs was not yet thirty, a bright legal mind with the potential to serve the ministry for decades, but already he'd been chucked out. Over the next decade he worked a little as a small-town lawyer but then more and more as a writer caught up in campaigning for German unification. Privately, he began to write to family members about his sexual desire for men, claiming that it was an "inherent" part of him. Under a pseudonym he began to publish pamphlets on the subject. Across two pamphlets in 1864, he introduced his idea of distinct categories: *urning*, or men who desire men; *dioning*, or people who are attracted to the opposite sex; and *urninden*, or women who desire women.

The following year he published three more pseudonymous pamphlets calling for tolerance and legal change. Although no law in Hanover formally punished same-sex acts, they were suppressed anyway by laws around public decency combined with prejudice, as Ulrichs himself had experienced at the ministry. His audacious pamphlets stirred up debates, and were distributed in Baden and Saxony, and even into Italy, France, the Low Countries and England. He also struck up a correspondence with Karl-Maria Kertbeny, another writer, who had begun to scribble anxious diary entries about fancying men.

Over the next five years, Ulrichs continued to develop his theories that same-sex desires were innate, and that gender and sexuality were interconnected. Among his ideas was the notion of a third gender, with the physical body of a man but the spirit of a woman – and made it clear that this was how he, the anonymous author, thought of himself. His friend Kertbeny wrote more and more on the subject too, in fact coining the words and concepts of *homosexualität* and *heterosexualität* as part of a person's nature.

Within this period, Prussia, which had laws against sodomy on its books, was also closing in on Hanover. This is when Ulrichs came to take a podium in Munich in 1867, at the sixth congress of the anti-Prussian Association of Jurists. It was an organisation that brought legal minds together to discuss, among other things, German unification, which it favoured. By 1867 they were on the back foot, with Prussia just having established the North German Confederation, and seeking to expand further. Ulrichs must have hoped that he could rely on the anti-Prussian sentiment in the room as he took to the stage to make an audacious argument.

The German states had laws causing innocent people to suffer and commit suicide, Ulrichs declared. Further expansion of Prussia would introduce an even harsher law against this group of innocents. When he revealed that he was talking about people who were drawn to members of the same sex, the shouting began. Cries from the crowd of five hundred lawyers included "Stop!" and "Crucify!" Ulrichs

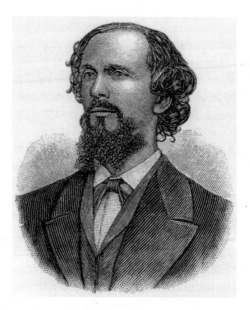

nearly stepped down, but a few curious minds encouraged him on. He told the room that the people he advocated for merely felt their desires as part of their nature. The speech was a sensation, but Ulrichs' case went nowhere.

He doubled down. The year after his speech, he published a pamphlet in which he described the experience of addressing such a hostile crowd. "I raised my voice in free and open protest against a thousand years of injustice," Ulrichs wrote – his words fierce, firm, and finally in his own name. "Unbiased, oral, and open debate of man-manly love has been until now kept under lock and key. Hatred alone has enjoyed freedom of speech. These barriers I have forcefully broken through – broken through without having offended thereby my duties to uphold public morality."

He titled the pamphlet *Raging Sword*, which surely should be adopted as a poppers brand name. The tract concluded with Ulrichs asserting a group identity, using the plural pronoun "we" to represent others like him. "We shall be steadfast," he promised. "We refuse further persecution."

The broader argument against Prussia had failed, and the state was expanding, swallowing up Ulrichs' native Hanover. In the preparations for revisions to the legal code, the Prussian Medical Affairs Board recommended against a sodomy law. Many of the nearly one hundred petitions to the Justice Minister also opposed it (five of them were from Ulrichs). Kertbeny opposed the law too, in two anonymous publications. But in May 1870 the law was promulgated. Paragraph 175 of the North German legal code outlawed sodomy, defining it as the sexual penetration of one man by another, and sexual conduct between man and beast. It would take one hundred and twenty-four years, until 1994, for this paragraph to be removed from German law entirely.

The anti-sodomy law came to pass despite Ulrichs' passionate advocacy. Looking at his actions now, I cannot help but think that he came from the future. Of course, as Ulrichs surmised, same-sex desire is timeless, simply part of human nature, mundane in its ubiquity. And yet the time and place where he found himself had converted attitudes into laws that did not accept it. He sought to resist and reform those laws, using language and argumentation. But more than a century would pass before the writer Audre Lorde would note that the master's tools will never dismantle the master's house.

So perhaps the reason why Ulrichs is a visitor to Hanover and Munich from the future is because of how he used himself, and his potential. He knew of his own body's pleasures, and felt confident enough in them to know that they were natural and not wrong. And so he let these feelings suffuse his legal arguments. He stood up in front of hostility and made a plea for pleasure. In his speech to his peers and his publications, Ulrichs became the first public advocate for the legal emancipation of queer bodies. He is described as "an improbable innovator" by Robert Beachy in his book *Gay Berlin*. The innovation he showed was really a performance. When he climbed onto the stage in a room filled with five hundred hot and bothered bodies, Ulrichs was a vision of freedom.

Two years after Ulrichs' failed appeal in Munich, Brunton arrived in Germany. Flush with the success of qualifying as a doctor and publishing innovative research on angina relief, he moved to Leipzig to deepen his research in a laboratory run by a scientist called Carl Ludwig. There, Brunton looked into the exact way amyl nitrite dilated blood vessels. Other researchers in different locations were also expanding humanity's knowledge of the smelly substance.

In the years that Ulrichs published pamphlets under his own name to call for legal reform for queer bodies, not very far away Brunton was furthering our understanding of what would become known as poppers. I like to imagine Brunton and Ulrichs crossing paths, perhaps at a bratwurst kiosk on a weekend break to Berlin, but actually Brunton did not stay long in Germany. He returned to London, and set up a laboratory of his own at University College. He also began to teach medicine at St Bartholomew's Hospital and continued to treat patients, alternating periods of focus on one side of his career or the other. He embodied his own belief that medicine could be better if doctors better understood how their therapies worked.

Through his career Brunton delivered on this potential. He became a therapeutic expert on the Pharmacopoeia Committee of the Pharmaceutical Society of Great Britain, a regular lecturer at the Chemists' Assistants' Association, and was named as a "great physician" in his obituary in the *Chemist and Druggist*, an industry newspaper, in 1916. "He had a wonderful charm with his patients," it reads, "and often his words did as much good as the medicine."[6]

Amyl nitrite continued to deliver on its own potential, too. When Brunton presented the substance to a meeting of the Pharmaceutical Society of Great Britain in December 1888, he "created much interest", according to a report in the *Chemist and Druggist*.[7] Use of amyl nitrite expanded through the medical profession, and other doctors began to try it out for all sorts of maladies. One such doctor was James Crichton-Browne, based in Yorkshire. He found amyl nitrite was useful for women, particularly in relieving menstrual cramps and the pain felt after childbirth. In seeing how it worked in patients, Crichton-Browne grew fascinated by the flushes it caused.

"In experimenting with the nitrite I have repeatedly noticed that whenever the flushing came out the patients grew stupid and confused and bewildered," he wrote in a letter dated April 16th, 1871. Crichton-Browne's correspondent was a scientist who was studying the biological aspects of human emotions, such as why we blush when we experience certain feelings. Crichton-Browne told his friend he would do anything to help the project, and sent him a stack of notes on his observations. The letter continued, "One woman who had the nitrite administered several times assured me, assured me [sic] that as soon as she got hot in the face she grew muddled all over."

The scientist who received that letter was Charles Darwin. It is not clear from Darwin's subsequent book whether he tried the amyl nitrite on himself or any subjects, even though Crichton-Browne advised him to: "Some experiments with this substance would I think throw valuable light on your researches, but they would require to be conducted with great care and caution, and would not be without danger."

Whether or not Darwin huffed, he definitely took an interest in Crichton-Browne's work. You can see why a scientist thinking about the emotional response of blushing would be interested in the physical response of flushing brought on by the sniffing of amyl nitrite. Darwin even wrote about amyl nitrite in *The Expression of the Emotions in Man and Animals* in 1872, citing his friend's work into how the flushing caused by sniffing amyl nitrite resembles blushing "in almost every detail".

Crichton-Browne's various recorded uses were also probably seen by the authors of Martindale, the entry in which for amyl nitrite described it as a "yellowish ethereal liquid with a peculiar and not disagreeable odour". The book lists amyl nitrite as being of use in the treatment of menstrual cramps and heavy bleeding after birth, as used by Crichton-Browne, but also asthma, migraine and even sea sickness. By 1883, when Martindale's pharmacopoeia was first published, amyl nitrite was still best known for angina, and its effectiveness had spread through the medical professions in other countries. An article in the *Boston Medical and Surgical Journal* described amyl nitrite as "the remedy par excellence for angina pectoris".[8]

A challenger to amyl nitrite had appeared, though. In 1879 William Murrell described his success in relieving the suffering of angina patients by giving them nitroglycerin. The substance had actually already been studied in animals, but it gave that original researcher such a bad headache that he did not want to try it in humans (that researcher was Brunton). Others persisted, and nitroglycerin actually came to take over amyl nitrite in the relief of angina. It is still prescribed in various forms today.

If you've ever done a pub quiz, you'll know that nitroglycerin is also the key ingredient in dynamite. This surprising use was patented in Germany by Alfred Nobel in 1867, the same year as the breakthroughs of our two body innovators. Ulrichs and Brunton's unconnected work in 1867 points to a queer future that neither man imagined. I am not saying that there is a particular date after 1867 when the queer future arrived. "Queerness is not yet here," wrote José Esteban Muñoz.[9] "We are not yet queer."

Muñoz wrote that in 2009 but in fact the date is irrelevant. He was claiming that queerness is forever out of reach. Muñoz is dead, along with Brunton and Ulrichs, and today queer peoples persist in finding new ways for our bodies to be, to perform, to fuck. Queerness is an attitude, our desire to challenge, to experiment in surprising ways. It is with this spirit of constant innovation that we must think about Ulrichs' speech and Brunton's discovery.

Many years passed before people began to sniff amyl nitrite while fucking each other. Brunton would surely have been surprised to see bottles of it passed around by gay men, one item among many in a sub-culture that also featured leather pants and coloured handkerchiefs. But I like to think that he would have welcomed gay men's experimentation, and their discovery of an alternative use for the stuff he popularised. He was a scientist, after all, and loved to study how substances interacted with the human body.

Ulrichs performed a future that every queerdo has to do, usually a thousand times – to declare, *this is who I am and there is nothing wrong with it*. No one had performed that rite before Ulrichs. It was a queer use of his body, and makes me think of the queer uses of our bodies that no one has yet performed. I think of both these men in the same way I think of bromine at room temperature. You cannot keep it down. It is an elemental force of nature that unsettles its surroundings – impassioned, reacting, forever seeking connection.

My body is knowable: pink skin, brown hair, two arms, two legs, penis, anus, inny belly button, that sort of thing. Symbols. I don't hear myself in "dude" or "bro". I am a man, for the paperwork, but there isn't a single thing in that word that marks it as a more specific category of "human". I hear myself in "gay", an echo down the centuries spoken by my sexually dissident elders. If I must use a word, I will use "queer" and be done with it. Will you look me in the eye, or what?

The labels declare a name for each small bottle. Jungle Juice, Everest, Blue Boy, Iron Horse, Double Scorpio, Oink!. Only symbols differentiate them. Typography, colour, design, illustration, trademarks, trade dress. The actual substances inside these bottles are obscured from us. Isoamyl nitrite, isobutyl nitrite, isopropyl nitrite, isopentyl nitrite. A technique called proton nuclear magnetic resonance spectroscopy can identify the mix of liquids inside each bottle. But the invisible vapour rising from them is the only thing that counts. "Iron Horse" is just a show.

When you unscrew their lids you smell their notes. You feel the effect pulse through you.

3. The Creation of Man?

Poppers, like man, were made in the USA. Every culture seems to create the categories of men and women and set certain standards for each. In some places, businesspeople convert these ideas into goods they can flog. This is the story of how, during the twentieth century, ideas about men, and gay men, were used to build poppers into a product that remains popular.

The story starts in the seventeenth century, when a ship landed in what is now the USA, carrying a family from what is now the Netherlands. Daughters Geertien and Sara, son Douwe, mother Hester Jans, and father Jellis Douw.[1] Their family name was Fonda, and in 1651 they settled in Fort Orange, now Albany, New York. The Fondas were among the eighty-two families who began to create a new life for themselves there, and indeed a new way of living entirely. The white settlers overtook Native American lands, and the Fonda family even established a village in their name on the site of the hamlet of Caughnawaga.

Jellis Douw Fonda distilled brandy, worked as a blacksmith, and became the patriarch of a North American dynasty. Fondas have proliferated far and wide in the USA. You can even track the growth of white power and expansion through the Fonda family. After Jellis Douw came gunstockers, farmers, soldiers, judges. By the turn of the twentieth century many of the Fondas were living in Nebraska. Among them was a baby boy called Henry, who would become one of the biggest stars in Hollywood, founding a dynasty of performing Fondas, through Jane and Peter and Bridget.

But it is another Fonda, born just a few years before Henry, whose story intersects with that of poppers. Howard Breese Fonda was born in 1896 to one of the Fonda families that had stayed east, in New Rochelle, New York. Howard would grow up to serve as a medic in the First World War, to build a career in pharmaceuticals, and even to invent an inhaler for sniffing amyl nitrite. His platform was Burroughs Wellcome, the pharmaceutical company that was already well known for finding ways to administer drugs. In the 1880s, the young outfit in London had grown by pioneering the sale of medicine in the form of tablets. By the time Howard came to work for the company in 1921, it had expanded internationally and opened a base of operations for North America in Tuckahoe, a village sixteen miles north of Manhattan.

This is where, not too far from where his Dutch ancestors had started their dynasty, Howard started as a medical representative at Burroughs Wellcome. At this time, amyl nitrite was manufactured and sold in glass ampoules. The ampoules were tiny cylindrical capsules, just a few centimetres long, tapered at one end into a seal forged by heat. Each ampoule contained a few millimetres of amyl nitrite in liquid form. They were sold for medical use, only under prescription, in small batches in branded tins. Patients suffering angina would be instructed to crush the glass of one ampoule and inhale the vapour released from the liquid inside. When the ampoule was opened in this way it made its famous "pop". The convenient distribution via ampoule had led to the kind of mass prescription that could only have been dreamt of by Thomas Lauder Brunton, when he had first used amyl nitrite on a patient with angina. Among other things, the fact that any single ampoule contained only a small volume of the stuff helped to avoid the kind of calamity that befell this poor girl in 1880:

She was ejecting great quantities of fluid from her stomach, which saturated the whole room with an amyl-like odour. Her face was grayish-white, her pupils widely dilated, her eyes glassy and vacantly rolling in their sockets. The mouth was wide open, breathing spasmodic and irregular.

This account was made by a doctor in Evansville, Indiana, after treating a young woman who had swallowed a dessert-spoon of amyl nitrite by mistake. His antidote was coffee, opium and a massage.[2] So ampoules were useful in preventing people like the Evansville girl from drinking amyl nitrite, but having to crush glass to release the vapour was not always safe. That is a problem Howard set out to solve.

Eleven years after Howard started at Burroughs Wellcome as a medical representative, he was appointed administrator of the research labs. Soon after, he became vice-president in charge of production. During this time, he developed a sophisticated device that would make amyl nitrite easier and safer to sniff. Although plenty of ampoules were already on the market, and used by various pharma companies in delivering amyl nitrite into patients' nostrils, Howard's would be contained in an inhaler.

In his patent application, filed on December 23rd, 1942, on behalf of his company, Howard claimed that his innovation protected the user from injury, prevented leakage of the contents, and could be manufactured at high quantities. It is a neat little object. The liquid is contained in an ampoule made from glass that is thin enough to be broken easily under pressure. The sealed ampoule is then wrapped in blotting paper, which spirals around the glass with diagonal gaps to allow for the escape of vapour once the glass is broken. Denser paper such as parchment creates an outer layer, also a spiral with gaps. When the patient squeezes the thing, the glass is crushed and the liquid spills into the blotting paper, which absorbs it. The parchment layer retains the glass fragments. The gaps in the paper spirals allow the vapour from the liquid to flow into the patient's hovering nostril.

Howard's patent application even notes that the paper could be coated with a substance that changed colour if the

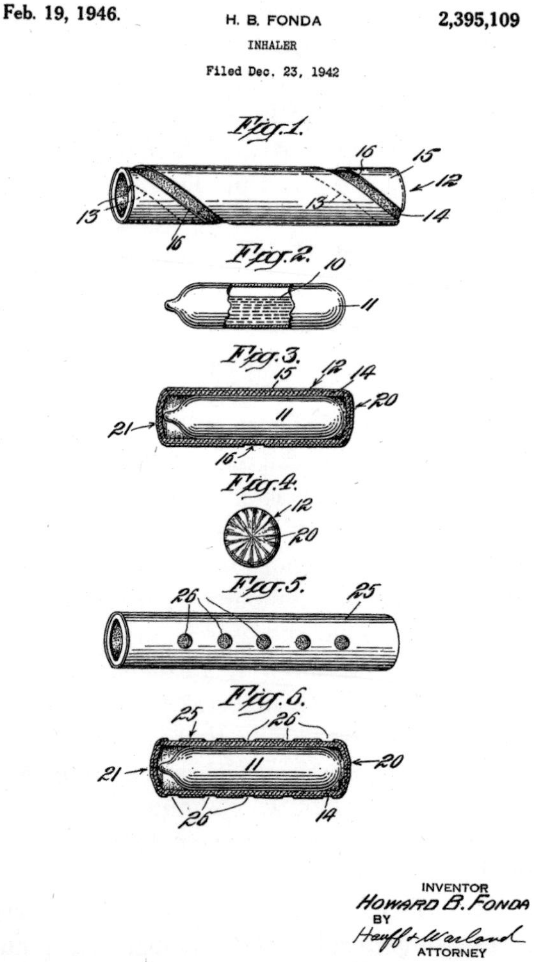

Feb. 19, 1946.   H. B. FONDA   2,395,109

INHALER

Filed Dec. 23, 1942

Fig.1.

Fig.2.

Fig.3.

Fig.4.

Fig.5.

Fig.6.

INVENTOR
HOWARD B. FONDA
BY
Hauff & Warland
ATTORNEY

liquid had leaked, so a person could spot a faulty ampoule. As an inventor he was thinking about the future and his lab descendants, noting breathlessly that "the invention is capable of various uses and that changes and modification may be made therein as will be readily apparent to a person skilled in the art". Howard continued in various executive roles at Burroughs Wellcome, which held the patent for his inhaler until it expired in 1963. Howard himself expired a year later.

If you read his obituary in the *Bronxville Review Press and Reporter*,[3] a local paper in upstate New York, you can see a through-line to Howard from the Fondas who arrived from what is now the Netherlands in the seventeenth century. It is the story of creating connections, building a name, working and living a respectable life. The article lists Howard's achievements, including his service to the military and to science, his success as a business executive, and as a family man. (It fails to mention his patent for a poppers inhaler.) Howard was survived by a widow, a son, a daughter and four grandchildren. After Howard, the Fonda family continued, as did his contribution to Burroughs Wellcome, which continues to live on inside the company that is now GlaxoSmithKline.

Howard Fonda is the kind of person that the USA created in the twentieth century: a businessman, an innovator, a husband, a father – a man in a smart suit on his way somewhere. There were few acceptable ways to be a man in Howard's golden era, roughly 1920 to 1960, but Howard seems to have adopted them. It is not hard to see Howard's life as being of a kind that many men aspired to in those years.

He could be Dan Brown in *The Hours*, the novel by Michael Cunningham. Although Dan is very much a peripheral character in a story focused on women, he is significant as a representative of what being a man was like.

He lives in the section of the novel set in 1949, and the reader gets to know him only through the eyes of his wife, Laura. It is her story really, an agonising exposition of being a housewife with a husband who does everything society thinks he should. Like Howard, Dan served in the military and now he works a steady job. All he wants is a contented family in a peaceful home. While Dan is the embodiment of settling down, Laura feels like she's missing out on another life. "Why did she marry him?" the book asks, and over the course of one day Laura finds her answer. "She married him out of guilt; out of fear of being alone; out of patriotism."

Laura walks around her perfect airy family home while Dan works at the office, trying to remind herself that it is a virtue to accept what you have. And yet she struggles with this ideal, especially in her husband. "Why does he desire nothing, really, beyond what he's already got?" He achieved the job, the wife, the house, the son – and that is enough. Laura yearns for more, which is why she drives herself to a motel room to sit and read *Mrs Dalloway* by Virginia Woolf.

The kind of turmoil that Laura feels inside is acted out in another novel set in the same period. But in *Revolutionary Road* by Richard Yates, the characters explode in anger. The man in this one is Frank Wheeler, who wants to appear likeable, interesting and exceptional. Like Dan Brown and Howard Breese Fonda, Frank served in the army. He believes he is destined for far greater things than sitting at a desk. He might not be pleased to admit to loving his office job at Knox Business Machines in New York City, but he does realise he is good at it. It is one of many paradoxes Frank has to live with in the suburban home he shares with his wife April.

April and Frank are drawn as monsters due to their circumstances. They act out their frustrations in not achieving greatness on each other. When she tells him she feels caught in a trap, Frank yells "don't make me laugh!" Later, when they make up after an argument, April apologises and makes the pledge he wants to hear. "And it seemed to him now that no single moment of his life had ever contained a better proof of manhood than that, if any proof were needed: holding that tamed, submissive girl and saying, 'Oh, my lovely; oh, my lovely,' while she promised she would bear his child."

But in another slanging match, April calls him self-deluded. She asks, "tell me how by any stretch... of the imagination you can call yourself a man!"

I'm thinking through the narrow ways that a male could think of himself in the USA in the 1940s and 50s. These fictional men are obviously symbolic. But I believe them to be accurate representations of what it felt like to be a middle-class man in the USA as business boomed, suburbia spread and bodies assembled into families. After the war had ended, this was how to build a future. But that vision relied on narrow ideas of what men could acceptably do. The characters in *The Hours* and *Revolutionary Road* wouldn't have suffered so much were it not for the idea of a man.

You only have to ask another Frank how narrow these expectations were. This Frank is real and in 1957 he was dismissed from his own steady job, as an astronomer in the US Army Map Service. Frank Kameny was fired for being gay, a condition that was deemed unfit for a public official. But Kameny's mistreatment upset the establishment more than his continued employment would have. That is because Kameny grew into one of the most important figures in the struggle for civil rights for gay people in the USA, protesting, litigating, lobbying and even running for office. His story echoes that of Karl Heinrich Ulrichs, with his campaign for gay rights after being forced to resign from his own government job in Hanover.

So Kameny was the kind of man who did not fit in with the Dan Browns and the Frank Wheelers or, perhaps, the

Howard Fondas. His performance of manhood was not acceptable to his employer, his government, or the majority of those he would describe as "my fellow Americans". In living an alternative kind of life, Kameny is among the many thousands of men who expanded what it could mean to be a man in the rich West, including perverting the very idea of it. Homosexuals like Kameny began to create a new kind of man from the middle of the century, and sometimes he could be found sniffing poppers when he was getting fucked.

It is impossible to pinpoint exactly when amyl nitrite became a recreational drug, and one used particularly by gay men to allay their inhibitions and intensify their orgasms. But it is safe to say that sphincters became well and truly relaxed in the 1960s.

In 1960, the US Food and Drug Administration (FDA) decided amyl nitrite was tame enough that the need for a prescription could be lifted. Patients suffering angina attacks could now obtain ampoules of amyl nitrite over the counter from pharmacists. But within four years, pharmaceutical companies were presenting evidence to the FDA that people were abusing their product. Pharmacists and pharmaceutical companies had noticed requests for amyl nitrite coming from healthy young men – not the usual demographic for angina. The pharma companies were nervous that either they or their customers could be harmed if their product was used for other purposes.

By the end of that decade, two men were on the Moon and many more were living gay lives in New York and San Francisco. These men were freer than ever, but they were still regularly intimidated with violence, including from police. In 1969, they joined other sexual and gender freaks in finally hitting back. The uprising at the Stonewall Inn expanded the homosexual rights movement that Kameny and others had been pushing for years, and gave it a fresh, angry and countercultural energy. In the same year, the FDA bent to the pressure from pharma companies and lobbyists concerned about amyl nitrite. The agency reinstated the need for a prescription. Of course, it was too late. Once you pop, you just can't stop.

Just as the New York Police Department had failed to stop queer people getting together to dance and fuck and live, the FDA failed to stop them sniffing poppers.

It is worth considering at this moment the competing ideas of what a man could be. By the late 60s, suburban Franks and Dans were still numerous, but they were definitely on the back foot. They were under attack from the proliferation of different ways to be a man, from hippies, Black Panthers, rebels, beatniks and poets. The booming sub-culture of perverts and queers in particular made things difficult for them too. Well-organised campaigners demanded the right for homosexuals to serve in government jobs and the military, and the removal of homosexuality from the psychiatrists' list of disorders in 1973. At the same time, pleasure-seeking queers lived their lives in defiance of what Dan Brown might have considered normal.

The Stonewall riot in 1969 had given gays the confidence to live more openly in their sexuality and gender presentation. The historian Jim Downs wrote in his book *Stand by Me* that the November 1970 issue of the magazine *Gay Sunshine* featured three naked men with shoulder-length hair and makeup, lounging on plush furniture. This was considered "feminine", but the representation in these images of the gay man in the early 1970s was positive and without the "shame" of femininity or weakness that had been thrown at gay men previously. That magazine was one of many created in the newly flourishing gay sub-culture. The suited campaigners for homosexual rights and their free-loving queer siblings together created newspapers, bookshops and cafes, churches and community groups. One thing that emerged from all this social innovation was a standard for how a gay man should look and behave, thanks to products sold for profit.

No committee decided that pecs and abs would become so dominant. That is not how capitalism works. It wasn't inevitable that hench guys would push aside the more swishy bodies on their plush furniture. But somehow through a combination of reproduction of this image, sexual desire, and social aspiration, the kind of man represented in Tom of Finland's drawings became king. According to Downs, he rose to power in the 1970s:

> No longer did [gay] newspapers focus on political and social issues. Now they published more and more flashy, glossy images of gay bodies. The macho clone appeared in newspapers, in ads for gay bars and bathhouses, on the covers of pornographic magazines, and in every other conceivable place that offered the opportunity for a sketch, photograph, or even cartoon image of a shirtless stud.

The Village People played up the alternative versions of this stud – think of their biker, builder, cowboy... each of that disco band's characters is a macho, macho man. They even made a song about him. "'Macho Man' from 1978 became the anthem of the new masculinity of the gay community," says Downs. Although gay life presented a challenge to patriarchy, somehow patriarchy came out on top again.

It is impossible to talk about the creation of this gay identity that has spread beyond America without acknowledging the little brown bottle in the room. Poppers were ubiquitous in the North American gay world. The poet Ian Young has written that poppers "became a staple of ghetto life, promoted almost exclusively through the commercial gay magazines and gathering-places".[4]

According to Young, "some disco clubs would even add to the general euphoria by occasionally spraying the dance floor with poppers fumes."[5]

Writing in the *Canadian Psychiatric Association Journal* in 1978, Stephen Israelstam, Sylvia Lambert and Gustav Oki say they visited homosexual bars, discotheques, and steam baths in Toronto and asked seventy people if they used poppers. No fewer than sixty-three had used them, usually twice a week. They concluded: "Their use is currently a craze amongst the male homosexual population."[6]

Poppers had only become more widely inhaled after the FDA's decision to reinstate the need for a prescription for amyl nitrite. That's because that substance was no longer the only way to get a poppers hit. The FDA decision had spurned innovators to synthesise similar substances that were untouched by regulation. Clifford Hassing, a medical student, was one such brainbox. He synthesised butyl nitrite in Los Angeles and named his concoction after its smell: Locker Room. Hassing's new poppers brand was a hit. He formed a company and began the industrial manufacture and sale of Locker Room. The market was competitive, especially as other street manufacturers began to tweak the traditional amyl nitrite into various substances. These were often marketed under the same brand names as amyl nitrite had been, but with labels that said they were "new and improved".

One ad for Locker Room poppers showed a butch superhero with a six-pack, cape and battering-ram thighs leaning against a locker door beside the words "Purity power potency". Another ad for Bolt poppers featured three guys, at least eighteen abs between them, one eagle tattoo and one motorbike, six side-burns and the gun from a gas pump dripping with fuel.

This Bolt ad was drawn by Rex, one of the most innovative, radical and influential artists of his generation.

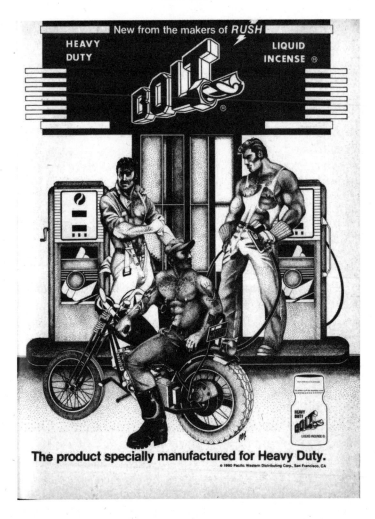

His work featured on bath house walls, nightclub posters and ads for phone sex – and it introduced a new way to see the sexualised male body. Rex's work appeared as part of an artistic movement of gay erotic art starting in the 1970s, that also included the photographer Robert Mapplethorpe and the artists Tom of Finland and Skipper. Poppers suffused these artworks. According to Jack Fritscher, who edited *Drummer* magazine, "Skipper told me he used poppers while drawing and painting his erotic pictures with one hand and masturbating with the other. 'Sniff. Have vision. Jerk. Jerk. Draw vision. Cum. Done.'"

Poppers brand names became just as testosterone-fuelled as the ad art, with the success in the 1970s of labels like Hard Ware and TNT (a wink to the shared birth year of dynamite and therapeutic amyl nitrite?). Slogans used phrases like "heavy duty", "the power you can count on", and "take off faster". These images, names and slogans drew on concepts that were associated with strength and the supposedly butch pursuits of fixing things or blowing them up. It can surely be no coincidence that humanity used these words and ideas connected with "being a man" to sell poppers at exactly the same time in human history that ideas of freedom blended with sexuality to form such a thing as a gay male identity. (I'm talking only in the rich world, especially North America.) Poppers were now a product, and very much a feature of gay dancefloors, bedrooms and cruising grounds.

What kind of man exactly was on offer to people who bought poppers? If you believed the ads, you would get a lot more than just a temporary lowering of blood pressure. The ads promised power and potency, the chance for one man to fuck another until their pecs exploded. Poppers manufacturers relied on the popularity of butch imagery from Tom of Finland and porn to advertise something as ephemeral as vapour that offers a brief head rush. It is remarkable how the advertising created a product – that product being the butch man who gays wanted to be, to possess, to fuck.

The magazine *Drummer*, aimed at men who liked to wear leather, championed what Fritscher called "homomasculinity". By 1978, the two most common words used by readers in their personal ads searching for a lover were "masculine" and "masculinity". (I don't know what these words mean exactly, but the users of gay dating apps who assert them today as desirable characteristics must have some grip on them.) Leathermen were very much a sub-culture within gay life in the USA and the UK at this time. They drew on ideas of working-class men from the straight world – breaking rank with the attempts of more academic or hippy types in New York to eliminate gender expectations and create an altogether new way of being a gay man. "Homomasculine identity was the key ingredient to *Drummer*'s success," Fritscher says in *Gay Pioneers*, his book about running *Drummer*, "because no one had anticipated, or affirmed, the unexpected news that masculine-identified gay men had to come out of the closet just like all the other gay identities."[7]

Take a moment to imagine the pathology of a gay man in the 1970s, born in the 40s or 50s, the era of Frank Wheeler and Dan Brown. Perhaps these characters were in fact the fathers of this gay man who made it to New York determined to escape suburbia and mandatory heterosexuality. He may have been rejected by his father Frank or his daddy Dan, disinherited, informed that he was considered a pervert and a degenerate. You cannot blame him for wanting to dance and drink and sniff poppers for a high that makes him want to be fucked into forgetting it all. Or to do that while wearing leather workers' boots and building his biceps. Whatever his show of gender, his aim was freedom. Poppers were just the potion.

The poppers sniffer is so different from Frank and Dan, and yet there are so many aspects of the man in the poppers ads that actual middle-class men like Frank and Dan aspired to. He is strong and potent, and he likes to work with his hands. In some ads, he is even a soldier, just like Frank and Dan used to be, depicted with dog tags and machine guns.

So although gay culture was creating a new kind of gay identity, it still relied heavily on conventional ideas of what it meant to be a man. Poppers were both countercultural, simply by being gay, and also deeply conventional in how they were marketed.

There are two big differences between the man represented by Dan and Frank, and the man represented in the poppers ads. The first is that poppers-man is sexualised, with exaggerated physical features and suggestive expressions. If you remove these characteristics from the ads, they could be selling engine oil to Dan in suburbia instead of peddling poppers to a disco queen in Manhattan. The second difference, by far more important, is babies. The barb inside April Wheeler's question of how Frank could by any stretch call himself a man is that he has not fathered a child. This is the main tension in their relationship. In contrast, Dan Brown is perhaps content because he has produced a child – a son no less. Only his wife wonders: is this all? Meanwhile Frank and April continue fighting over their dreams and their decisions as they remain childless. A kind of peace falls when April says yes, she will bear a child. The promise of fatherhood is the thing that gives Frank a momentary happiness. With a child his picture will be complete – even though it was not a picture he previously wanted. Frank is convinced that he is exceptional, that he could have been something. As he comes to realise this may not be the case, perhaps the unborn child gives him a shot at a legacy, a way to project himself into the future.

Dan has a child in the bag already, but he could not know that his little Richie would grow up to join the Stonewall generation of poppers-sniffing disco-gays. This generation, freed from suburbia, did not seem interested in the future at all. Tonight was all that mattered. They didn't do the kind of sex that created babies, and nor were they interested in finding a way to have a baby. Gay people today are asked if they want to have children simply because they can, as long as they can afford it (through adoption, surrogacy, co-parenting). But their ancestors in the 1970s were not thinking about that. If they thought about the future at all, they thought about tomorrow's hangover.

Let there be no negative judgement about this hedonism. A desire for pleasure right now is no sin. And it certainly made the gay man distinct from other men in the USA in the 1970s. The pleasure principle, and specifically the openly acknowledged one of gay sex, was a novel way to be a man. But in so many other ways, as seen in the marketing of poppers, even these gay men were driven by much more mainstream desires: to work a trade or fight a war and to always be strong.

In any case, some people thought all the hedonism was getting to be too much. Although Pete Fisher was a gay liberation activist, he ended up writing a novel called *Dreamlovers* that looked back with some degree of alarm at a fictionalised version of himself in the 1970s. Fisher's lover in the book urges him: "Enjoy yourself as much as possible. Get into pleasure." Writing about this book, Young says, "Pleasure for gay men was now the porn-and-poppers lifestyle. Fisher, whose two great joys in life are his writing and his lover, is confused, but not wanting to be possessive or rigid, he goes along."[8]

The obsession with pursuing pleasure in such uniform ways became a parody of itself: gays began to describe themselves as clones. Perhaps the best description of this sub-sub-culture, its symbols and its pathology, was given by a woman called Alison Henegan, a writer, thinker and editor. She was also a consultant on *Gay Life,* the first British television programme that was made by gays and lesbians. In one episode, Henegan appeared as a talking head thinking aloud about gay male identity. Through her glasses and down her nose, Henegan informed the British public in 1980:

One of the fastest growing new looks is the clone look, which came to us by courtesy of New York, and is threatening to take over... The little tash, and the shirt, and the jeans and the boots, and a certain look of controlled, mean, innate superiority, which you can see on the floor of any disco that you're unwise enough to enter. I suppose if you're an advocate of that look you'll see it as utterly to be applauded because it's totally ordinary. And if you're less happy you'll see it as a lemming-like drive to total uniformity which makes you think that gay men apparently come in batches of one hundred.[9]

So the USA in fact made several men in the twentieth century. First came men like Dan: the post-war family man. He looked up to strong and straight male characters like the leads in *The Grapes of Wrath* (1940) and *Mister Roberts* (1955), both played by Henry Fonda.

Second, the faggot. By pathologising and persecuting gay men, such as Frank Kameny, US culture made him into an "other", and a distinct category of man was born. But the occupants of this category took control of it, fighting back, claiming their rights, and becoming the third type of man, the liberated faggot. The final step was the emergence from within that category of the beefcake who wants to fuck and be fucked, and look muscly all the while.

Ads for poppers promised that a man could become this beefcake simply by sniffing nitrites. Of course that was a false claim, but really the purpose of the ads was to promote consumption. The standard ideas of men who were admired within liberated gay culture, from the beefcake to the clone (barely a hair between them, really) were always uniform, with certain standards of beauty, clothing, behaviour. Almost all of them overlapped with mainstream aspirations in the USA for being a man that Frank and Dan would have recognised (although they may have turned away from the sexualisation). This is why Henegan was so filled with despair by 1980 when she surveyed the dancefloor and found only butch lemmings. She might be just as sad today, in the 2020s.

Although there are many more poppers brands than ever before, they often try to make themselves sound manly: Hulk, Black Tiger, Fist, Iron Horse. Even Bolt and Hard Ware are still going strong. It is possible in the 2020s to consume these products with irony. But the spreadsheets in the companies that make them log only sales. There is no column for ironic sales. The enduring success of marketing poppers in this way suggests that something persists in the aspiration towards an idealised manhood.

Poppers may have been the first body products to use butch tones to sell themselves to men. Today shop shelves are filled with Mancave grooming gear, Bulldog beard oil and Sport Impact shower gel. "That's not a flavour, that's a concept," sings Mawaan Rizwan in his song "Mango", "I don't wanna wash myself in a concept." But Rizwan and the rest of us are awash in the concept of "man". The USA keeps manufacturing him, in products, in films, in gym adverts. Politicians still try to appeal to the idea of the family man who descends directly from Frank and Dan. And gay culture still reproduces bulging pecs and seductive power in its promotional images for gay club nights around the world. You might want to reject the dominant ideas of what it means to be a man, but we are constantly reproducing him.

As a teenager I used to buy second-hand CDs from eBay, which always arrived in those envelopes that are padded with bubble wrap. This is how I grew my music library and had my first hands-free orgasm.

Wedging a padded envelope between my mattress and the box-spring of my bed made a hole that was penetrable but tight under the weight of the mattress. Petroleum jelly was spread inside for lubrication, porn printed out from the internet and laid on the bed. Knees on the floor, eyes on the images, my dick pushing inside.

Neither the envelope nor the jelly were designed for this precise use. And as a teenager I was realising that my body was not designed at all. Curious, searching, testing. A body is open by nature, solid but also mostly fluid.

4. Sex / Death

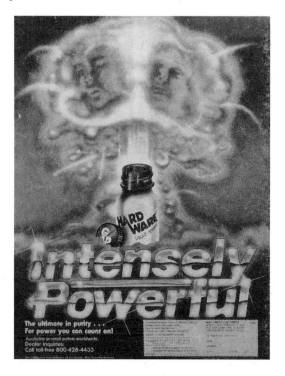

The words "Intensely powerful" sparkle in metallic silver. Atop them sits a bottle of Hard Ware poppers with its lid off. A vapour is rising, actually *shooting* from the opening, coalescing into a mushroom cloud. It is the kind of cloud created by the atomic explosion that murdered as many as 146,000 people in Hiroshima in 1945. Men's euphoric faces can be seen in the detail of the amassing vapour. If you step back from the image, the cloud as a whole looks like a human skull. "The ultimate in purity" is the slogan printed underneath, beside a toll-free phone number for more information about Hard Ware poppers.

This ad ran in 1981 in *Drummer*, a magazine for gay men into leather and sado-masochism. It is hard to know exactly what is going on in the mushroom cloud of pleasure and annihilation, but sex and death are often linked in our imaginations, as advertisers know. You can avoid the ultimate come-down simply by purchasing their wonderful, life-affirming products. Cosmetics, vitamin pills, fast cars, salads, yoga mats – this is how to feel alive. But as the ad for Hard Ware poppers shows, advertisers for gay products have long had to do something more distinctive, by sexualising men, glorifying death, or both.

Looking back at the hedonistic gay 1970s, the combination of subversive codes and sexual ones seems inevitable. Through that period, gay men amassed in places like London, New York and San Francisco. They lived together, but also apart from homophobia as much as they could. They fucked a lot. It is common for stigmatised people who are suffering psychological pain through harassment and discrimination to join together. Through bath houses, cruising guides, nightclubs and magazines like *Drummer*, a sub-culture of gays moved closer and closer, and deeper and deeper into sex. Every sub-culture needs its opium. Use of poppers boomed.

But sniffers wanted to know whether their quick high was damaging. It was hard to find this out, because use remained limited primarily to men having sex with men. In rich countries like the USA and the UK, although such men were increasingly liberated, their lives were still misunderstood and furtive. It is not hard to imagine gay people remaining cagey about their drug use and sex lives, as the politicians were decrying them and the police were rounding them up. It is also not hard to imagine that harm could be caused by a product with a dubious legal status that advertisers and vendors could not tell consumers how to use. In 1976, the USA's National Institute on Drug Abuse recorded emergency room admissions resulting from nitrite side effects – but only thirteen.[1]

Still, the uncertainty about this relatively old drug with this relatively new use gave some people pause. Although every substance interacts with our bodies as well as our minds, poppers in particular raised some fascinating concerns, such as whether they could damage your heart. Users needed advice.

From 1974 onwards, in the UK, if you spoke English and you wanted to know anything about the lives of gay people or lesbians, you phoned a room in the basement of a bookshop on Caledonian Road in London. In this room, all day and all night, every day of the year, sat the volunteers of Gay Switchboard. To callers, this was a simple non-judgmental service giving out information about club nights and sex positions, as well as emotional support to those who felt isolated and rejected by homophobic society. The helpline was just another feature of a booming queer sub-culture. But in the unmarked room beneath a store of radical, leftist books, Gay Switchboard grew into a sophisticated operation. It took over a bigger space above the shop, where volunteers built shelves and shelves to hold bursting information files, developed a detailed training programme on how to handle any type of call, and laid down a culture of internal debate on how to respond to callers' needs.

Almost as soon as they began taking calls, volunteers were talking about poppers. Their primary offer here, as with every other topic raised on calls, was supplying information such as where to get hold of them. But the log books at Gay Switchboard also record a range of opinions about them. "People who sniff poppers need an extra physical kick from sex as they get no emotional satisfaction," wrote one volunteer, David Seligman, on August 29th, 1975, in his characteristic all-caps handwriting. An anonymous colleague responded on the same day: "You sanctimonious tie-wearer."[2]

It may seem surprising that this dispute existed at all. Gay Switchboard sat at the heart of what we now might call London's queer politics. Indeed, it was co-founded by people who graduated from an intense few years of activism in the Gay Liberation Front. It was housed in the same building as other radical projects trying to lever Britain out of its conservatism. But Gay Switchboard was a broad church, comprising Christians such as Dudley Cave and tie-wearers like Seligman, who were responsible for keeping the organisation going, alongside hippies and radicals. A few days after Seligman's claim that poppers were for people who lacked emotional satisfaction from sex, a volunteer called George responded. "I've had emotional and physical pleasure heightened by occasional use of poppers," wrote George, "and I would think that anyone who asks should be told that there's no harm in them, unless you have a dodgy heart."[3]

These exchanges were recorded in ink in the phoneroom at Gay Switchboard in 1975. Perhaps this moment was when gay men began to divide themselves into those who pursued pleasure and those who pursued marriage.

Seligman deserves to be remembered as a man who saved and improved countless lives through his work with Gay Switchboard. The project became a hugely important charity that still takes calls today as Switchboard – the LGBT+ Helpline. Today's volunteers would not imply that sex brings either emotional or physical satisfaction, and yet Seligman's idea persists broadly in society. There are few acts derided as much as "meaningless sex" – it is a term that people disdain on dating apps as they proclaim an orientation towards a long-term relationship. Many of us share the idea that the less sex you have, the more meaningful it will be. This is one reason why we place so much pressure on ourselves when we have sex, after a break from it, or in the case of waiting for a first time.

By the 1970s gay sex was defiant, and more associated with pleasure and alternative living than the suburban monogamous heterosexuality that so many queer ancestors had endured. Gay sex in particular was enhanced by poppers, especially among men. Fucking became a new way of life. And yet, in 1981, many of the men who lived in this way began to die, fast and horribly.

"Present indications are that we are seeing a truly new syndrome," wrote David T. Durack in the *New England Journal of Medicine* in December of that year.[4] Men seen by doctors like Durack had turned up to hospitals with a range of problems. Purple lesions grew on their bodies, caused by an unusual cancer. As Durack wrote, five or six new cases of this Kaposi's sarcoma were appearing each week. He also logged an outbreak of a kind of pneumonia rarely seen in people who were otherwise young and fit. The men struck down with these rare diseases were all having sex with men, prompting Durack to ask: Why this group? Why now, and not before?

He suspected something new was compromising these men's immunity. "Fashions in drug use change frequently, and experimentation with new agents is common," wrote Durack. "Perhaps one or more of these recreational drugs is an immunosuppressive agent. The leading candidates are the nitrites, which are now commonly inhaled to intensify orgasm." This is how the connections began to form between poppers, gay sex and the patients with these unusual sicknesses.

In 1982, three doctors, T.J. McManus, L.A. Starrett and J.R.W. Harris, wrote a letter to the *Lancet* to say that they had asked 250 male homosexuals visiting their clinic in St Mary's Hospital in London if they had inhaled nitrites, and 86% said yes.[5] The number was the same in New York, San Francisco and Atlanta, according to a special report published in the same year in the *New England Journal of Medicine*. The London doctors wrote: "Similarities, therefore, exist between the recreational habits of male homosexuals in London and those of homosexual males living in areas of the USA where the immunocompromise syndrome has been found."

By spring 1983, the BBC was projecting images of poppers bottles into living rooms across the UK. The broadcaster's first documentary on what became known as AIDS and the human immunodeficiency virus that caused it was called *Killer in the Village*.[6] The programme featured a New York doctor, Alvin E. Friedman-Kien, handling a dozen poppers bottles and reading off their brand names in a voice that tried to sound like scientific objectivity. He said that of his patients suffering from the new illness, 100% had used poppers. Following the same approach as the scientific literature at the time, the programme left the correlation hanging.

The film also featured the back of a man's head as he talked about poppers. The narrator introduced this man as the president of New York Gay Men's Health Crisis and said he had chosen to remain anonymous on the programme "to avoid problems in his job". At the time, that position was held by Paul Popham, a high-profile gay rights activist. The anonymous contributor was almost certainly Popham. In the programme, he showed another doctor, Linda Laubenstein, how to sniff poppers. She looked a little sheepish, glancing at someone off camera before turning back to ask, "How long does a bottle like that last?" The contributor told her that it would be passed around from person to person at a disco and wouldn't last beyond one night.

The programme raised far more questions than it answered, and it terrified many queer people who saw it. "It said AIDS was a disease for which there was no treatment or cure, which was fatal, and it was something which you could catch from having sex with an American," said a contributor to *The Log Books* podcast, who was sixteen when he watched the documentary.[7] "I'd just had sex with an American, and I thought, I'm fucked."

All the documentary could do was repeat the questions of scientists and clinicians, making correlations between gay life and the "killer disease". One scene combined images of the gay districts of Los Angeles with narration claiming that as many as 400,000 gay men had congregated there in recent years due to greater sexual openness. The voice asks, "Did this contribute to the spread of AIDS?" The dream that gay sex was a valid way to live was turning into a nightmare. Suddenly, it was a way to die. In the public imagination the *category* of being gay became linked to death, in common tabloid phrases such as "gay plague" and "gay killer bug". Really HIV is transmitted through particular sex acts, as well as non-sexual acts such as intravenous drug use, done by all sorts of people, and yet it was the label "gay" that stuck and had a huge impact in how the disease was viewed. This was not at all inevitable.

As it became clear how men having sex with men were affected, their bodies were seen as belonging to a distinctive category and their behaviours were scrutinised. AIDS bled from science documentaries and the gay press into a major story on the nightly news, where all sorts of correlations were made. One piece of research covered broadly was a study by Harry Haverkos, a doctor at the National Institute of Allergy and Infectious Diseases in the USA.[8] He had looked at eighty-seven AIDS patients and compared the ones who had Kaposi's sarcoma with those who developed pneumonia or other diseases. He found that those with

Kaposi's sarcoma used poppers the most.

"Kaposi's sarcoma is a cancer of blood vessels, and nitrites cause the blood vessels to dilate," Haverkos is quoted as saying in a story in the *Washington Post* about his research on April 24th, 1985. "So you have the product having an effect in roughly the same place you're getting the cancer." He makes it sound like a decent guess. As people looked into gay sex and this awful illness, searching for causation, poppers looked like a prime suspect.

HIV and AIDS caused a crisis: health, housing, politics, heartbreak. In the centre of this, in the USA, were two men – activists John Lauritsen and Hank Wilson. They were both watching men around them getting sick and dying. The US government was ignoring the epidemic and many people were unsympathetic to a group of people who they already viewed as disgusting. Wilson and Lauritsen had been working separately on gay rights for years. In San Francisco Wilson had campaigned against the discrimination of gay teachers. And from New York Lauritsen was writing articles about the epidemic, including challenging researchers for claiming that the thing called AIDS was caused by an infectious agent (which, ultimately, it is).

When the correlations between AIDS and poppers came out, Wilson and Lauritsen were concerned. They were shocked that no one in the gay world was sounding an alarm, so they decided to collaborate. They first published a pamphlet aimed at educating gay men about these correlations, and then founded a campaign called the Committee to Monitor Poppers. It was probably not really a true committee, since the only two names ever associated with it were Wilson and Lauritsen's. The group was registered at 55 Mason Street in the Tenderloin district in San Francisco, the address of the Ambassador Hotel that Wilson was running as a kind of hospice for people living with AIDS.

In 1986, they published *Death Rush: Poppers and AIDS*,[9] a short book that synthesised research, reporting and the authors' loud pleas for their fellow gays to put down the little brown bottle. "Giving up poppers would seem, at least in the beginning, like giving up sex itself," they wrote. "With regular use, they become a sexual crutch, and many gay men are incapable of having sex, even solitary masturbation, without the aid of poppers."

Lauritsen and Wilson were convinced that poppers were implicated in causing AIDS. "The question is no longer *whether*, but rather *how much* of a role... Are poppers a relatively minor or a very major co-factor?" Most sections in the book ended with either loaded questions like this, or declarations like "the only sane course of action is to stop using poppers immediately".

In *Death Rush*, you can hear the fear in Wilson and Lauritsen's words. Although manufacturers fought back with PR and lobbying, the alarm was heard in Washington, DC. The Anti-Drug Abuse Act of 1988 named butyl nitrite, one of the common substances in poppers, as a "banned hazardous product". The law explicitly stated that butyl nitrite was not to be used in commercial products "for inhaling or otherwise introducing it into the human body for euphoric or physical effects".[10] This was a tiny part in President Ronald Reagan's so-called war on drugs, which among other things, created the policy goal of a drug-free USA.

On a wave of victory, Lauritsen took his words to the UK, writing an article for the London-based *Capital Gay* newspaper on March 31st, 1989. His only quoted source was his friend and collaborator Wilson; the article was an opinion piece by a campaigning journalist suddenly on the winning side. "No longer can poppers be presented as harmless 'room odourisers', or as an accepted part of the gay male lifestyle," he wrote. He was wrong, of course.

Sticking to the letter of the law, manufacturers and sellers continued to do the exact thing Lauritsen said was no longer possible: describing poppers as harmless household product. They printed labels with "room odouriser" or "leather cleaner", as they had been used to doing anyway, and sometimes added "not for human consumption". The problem with prohibition is people.

The US ban worried some sellers in the UK though. The landlord of the Market Tavern gay pub in Nine Elms, London, stopped selling poppers from behind the bar,[11] no doubt others were just as cautious. But the canny editors of *Capital Gay* must have wanted to assure their readers who enjoyed poppers. Alongside Lauritsen's article they included their own text, ostensibly to introduce Lauritsen to a UK-based audience. But the note also pointed out that poppers were not banned in the UK, and indeed Joseph Miller, owner of the biggest poppers company in the USA, was looking to expand production into Europe.

Poppers makers were not taking no for an answer. They must have known two things. First, any good news for the anti-poppers campaign in the USA was just the halo effect of ever stricter actions against drugs and crime. On top of the 1988 act that banned butyl nitrite, the Crime Control Act of 1990 banned the broader category of alkyl nitrites, which included other poppers substances.[12] This bill's sponsor was Joe Biden, Democrat senator from Delaware, who became president in 2021. The new ban just meant that, in order to remain lawful, poppers made from other nitrites, not just butyl, had to carry labels either saying they were not for human consumption, or that they were room odouriser.

Second, Lauritsen was losing ground with his claim, which he made again in the *Capital Gay* article, that there were "strong epidemiological links between the development of AIDS and especially Kaposi's sarcoma". It had become clear that HIV was the cause of AIDS-defining illnesses, and that HIV was transmitted through sex. Poppers, like alcohol and other drugs, can lower inhibitions and encourage the user into more sex, but that is the only known connection to HIV.

But because it became more widely known that HIV/AIDS cases often involved two men, anal fucking, and sometimes poppers, people began to see sex as much as a problem as the virus itself. Deviant sex plus death can cause an explosion. This is how the public conversation about the epidemic became one about morality.

By 1986, the moral debate had bled into the scientific one. Speaking on a British documentary called *AIDS: A Strange and Deadly Virus*,[13] the US animal virologist Opendra "Bill" Narayan represented the concerns over gay men's sex lives, especially their promiscuity. "These people have sex twenty to thirty times a night," he said on the programme. "A man comes along and goes from anus to anus and in a single night will act as a mosquito transferring infected cells on his penis. When this is practiced for a year, with a man having three thousand sexual intercourses, one can readily understand this massive epidemic that is currently upon us."

We now know that HIV is actually harder to transmit than Narayan implied, but really it is not the bad science that makes this contribution so awful. It is the moral tone. The documentary was from the BBC Horizon series, the same as the one mentioned earlier, from 1983. In that earlier one, the clinicians, researchers and producers remained curious about AIDS, as well as alarmed. By 1986, as Narayan showed, morality had crept in. The twin fears of sex and death hampered any chance of a humane response to the illness.

In the same year, the chief constable of Greater Manchester, James Anderton, said that homosexuals, drug addicts and prostitutes who had HIV/AIDS were "swirling in a human cesspit of their own making". For this, he was named Bigot of the Year 1987 by readers of *Capital Gay* newspaper,[14] a title he took from the prime minister, Margaret Thatcher, who won the award in 1986. She gave Anderton a good run for the award in 1987, though, rejecting calls for a public inquiry into Anderton's conduct and writing a letter supporting him.

Thatcher's actions were the result of her brilliant ability to divine whatever is considered "public opinion". Even if most of the population in Britain may not have spoken as inhumanely as Anderton, Thatcher must have known that most people agreed with him. There is always moral sex and immoral sex, and it was clear in the 1980s as gay men were dying that many people thought gay sex was bad. This moral atmosphere forced every single individual to make their own decisions.

For some, the only choice was abstinence. "Large numbers of people have become chaste, are no longer seeking sexual satisfaction with other people, period," said Bobby Campbell, a man living with HIV, in *Killer in the Village*. Later in the documentary a sexual health counsellor chatted to two guys on the street about AIDS. "How do you get it?" they asked. "Is there a cure for it? Can they put a stop to it? Medicine?"

They seemed to have been stopped in the street as they went about their young, carefree business. One of them was holding a can of Coke, the other was wearing shades. They looked incredibly shocked when the counsellor told them the new disease had no cure, could kill within a year, and was transmitted through sex. "That's tough," said one of the guys. Told that his chances of contracting it would increase with his number of sexual partners, he said, "Yes, I would stop having sex." His friend added, "Oh, definitely."

Because we fear death, HIV/AIDS made us fear sex. Even the generation of gay men who had fucked through the 1970s, helping to create radical new ways of relating and living and enjoying their bodies, became scared of sex. That is of course understandable: HIV and the AIDS-related illnesses are horrible, and seeing your friends and lovers die is a trauma. It would be wrong to make any judgement on any individual's choice to avoid sex, given these circumstances. But it's sad that many of them enacted exactly what conservatives wanted: an end to gay sex. In the USA, William F. Buckley was the loudest, arguing in newspaper columns that people living with HIV should be tattooed with their status and undergo forced sterilisation. In the UK, Tony Gifford, also known as the third Earl of Halsbury, decried gays in parliament for their "disgusting and unnatural practices like buggery". He said, "They act as reservoirs of venereal diseases of all kinds."

Halsbury's words were made as he proposed a bill to peers that would stop local authorities buying children's books featuring same-sex families, and other forms of "promotion of homosexuality". In support of Halsbury's bill, Frank Pakenham, also known as the seventh Earl of Longford, said, "Homosexuals, in my submission, are handicapped people... In so far as an attempt is being made to expand homosexualism throughout this community, the outcome can only be fatally disruptive for the family."[15]

Traditionalist voices like these used the atmosphere of fear caused by HIV/AIDS to campaign against any way of living beyond a traditional family model. There are two things going on here: first, an incorrect assumption that a "family" only constitutes a man and a woman and their own conceived children; and second, that the sex that takes place outside of this model, especially bum fun between two men, is therefore destructive, harmful and dangerous. Throw in HIV and their sex also becomes fatal.

These twin fears of sex and death pre-dated HIV/AIDS, but they are left darker by that crisis. The epidemic, which is an ongoing catastrophe in many places, has also made us scared of what sex-related substances can do to our bodies. This is what one commentator wrote when a new drug came onto the market in 1998 that could help men to have sex: "It is precisely among drug abusers that Viagra's potential for harm looms largest," wrote Gabriel Rotello in the *Advocate* on July 7th of that year. "Crystal meth in particular makes its users sexually voracious but impotent – a world of bottoms searching for a top. The epidemiological effect of a drug that, in the words of one crystal meth user, 'turns every bottom into a top as well', could really give HIV transmission a nasty boost."[16]

The fear that Viagra would lead to more gay sex that spreads disease did not endure. But concern over poppers returns to the public debate every so often. In 2017, the worry became eye damage, thanks to a widely publicised study from researchers at the Sussex Eye Hospital and the University of Lincoln.[17] The researchers found evidence among twelve men that using poppers had caused the deterioration of their foveas, the part of the eye responsible for the clearest parts of our vision. Specifically, it was the poppers brands that contained isopropyl nitrite that caused the problems, although the research did not manage to understand exactly how. All the patients recovered their vision when they stopped using poppers, but the finding still made some users nervous. If blindness, why not also death?

Poppers have caused some deaths, mostly from drinking the substance. Every few years a story like Jacob Langford's appears, as a reminder of how deadly poppers can be. In 2018, Jacob was a twenty-two-year-old man who went to the Rainbow Serpent music festival in western Victoria in Australia. You only have to read the online tributes to know how much this young chef and skateboarder loved living and how much people loved to share his life with him. But Jacob died at the festival. Sixteen substances were found inside his body, including ketamine, cocaine, diazepam, Xanax, MDMA, MDA, temazepam, oxazepam, atropine and alcohol. This combination would have been enough, of course. But the thing that tipped him over was when he swallowed the contents of a bottle of poppers.

Jacob's friends yelled at him to vomit, but he collapsed. As the medics tried to save him, they could smell amyl nitrite on his breath. "No one should be taken this young," wrote one mourner on a crowdfunder page made to help Jacob's family. "You will always be at rainbow in spirit," wrote another. "The land is magical and you are blessed to be able to stay at rainbow as long as the festival continues. And beyond. Mad love."

A story like Jacob's churns the stomach. He sought joy, and found death. These connections between poppers, sex, sickness and death reveal something dark about the reality of living in our bodies: many of us are scared that our pleasures will end and our bodies will die. Our minds cannot seem to help linking sex and death – even when that link is bizarre, as in the case of the poppers advert with the atomic cloud that opened this chapter. Advertisers know that sex sells, but shock and fear can sell harder. The Hard Ware advert implies that the intensity of the pleasure you'll feel when you sniff the product is matched by the intensity of suffering in a nuked city. Only the USA would annihilate thousands *and also* produce art connecting this catastrophe to sexual ecstasy in an advert for a bum-opening product labelled as "intensely powerful".

The people behind that advert pushed the boundaries of taste and sensitivity because they knew how we think about sex and death. We link them – at least unconsciously, which is the realm where adverts do most of their work.

Imagine a horizontal line with sex at one end and death at the other. The experience of living sits in the middle of the line, and it is where we spend most of our healthy days. In our moments of sex, our bodies feel like they have moved beyond mere living. Done well, sex can feel like the opposite of death. Done among a community of similarly maligned people, it can feel like a shared future. But the story of poppers is not only about how they relieve suffering and enhance pleasure. It is about how they bend the line, how sex and death seem to reach for each other, how sex and poppers were blamed for death, and how an extreme pleasure tastes like dying.

Perhaps there is something else too: some of us are scared of those who enjoy certain types of sex. Seligman is not the only person ever to believe in physical sex and emotional sex as two distinct categories. Many of us make a negative judgement on sex that is driven more by touch than feeling. I am not even sure how to make the distinction, but plenty of us manage it. And lots of people also believe some sex belongs in a cesspit, or even that it can be unlawful even if consensual, as in the case of the British police who arrested men having sex with each other in public toilets and parks. Others still believe gay sex in particular is wrong because it sits outside of an idealised family construct.

So there is always moral sex and immoral sex. At its worst, sex is seen to cause disease and death. This isn't true; AIDS-related illnesses like Karposi's sarcoma take hold under the condition of poor immunity, which is a result of an attack by the human immunodeficiency virus. But of course it is true that you increase your risk of contracting this virus the more sex you have with different people. So moral sex is sex that is infrequent, done with one other only, and makes a family or has the chance of doing so. It is also disease-free. All of these things are about the future, about living longer and healthier – as an inherent good. And they mean you can live even beyond your own future, with your genes replicating through your children and other future generations. Preferably moral sex is more about emotional connection than physical pleasure too, for many people. This gives it more meaning, whatever that means.

There is an alternative to all this – sex for fun, sex for now, sex as an emotional and physical experience at the same time. Call it queer sex – sex that doesn't care about creating families, or categories, or even relationships that are seen as acceptable. Call it fearless sex – sex between people who know that it is things like viruses and bacteria, not sex, that cause disease. Call it feeling sex – because sex contains both physical and emotional experiences. Even simply wanting to fuck is an emotion.

We take sex far too seriously. We agonise instead of enjoy. We measure more than we pleasure. We judge how others do it, when we might better spend our time wondering what we might learn from them. We also pretend that sex is everything else but sex, by converting fast cars, deodorant, salad, even poppers *into* sex in order to sell these products. Films depict sex far less than they do extreme violence, and yet sex is much more a part of our lives. When you compare the things we produce that are sex-y (that is, about sex) with the actual sex that you are familiar with, it all seems completely bizarre – as with that Hard Ware ad that promises an orgasm at the same time as a nuclear catastrophe.

There is another way to read that silly ad. It is so ridiculous that perhaps it is fun. The makers certainly know how good sex can feel, especially with a sniff of Hard Ware. And if the dominant treatment of sex is to fill it with significance, then here is an alternative: sex that is fun, fearless, feeling and queer. Any sex coming close to these is something to desire. Sometimes it's hard to know whether we are more afraid of death, or of sex.

You dye your hair.

You inject testosterone so we can all see the real you.

Your heart is induced into its beats by a pacemaker.

Clomipramine keeps you believing.

You take an estrogen and a progestogen because you don't want a baby.

I sniff isoamyl nitrite so I can feel extra pleasure when I touch myself, or when you penetrate me, or when we kiss and dance and love. Are any of these things necessary? Do I behave differently because of this intervention? If you can spare the money, or you live in a country with a certain set of priorities, you can take a daily tablet of emtricitabine and tenofovir that stops HIV multiplying if it enters your blood. I think about that too. If HIV is what I worry about, I can take the tablet and forget condoms, forget the pause, forget the decision, the terror. I can be the free spirit my ancestors dreamed of as they lay dying.

We wear frames fitted with lenses so we can see the world.

5. Utopia for a Moment

You are watching the drag queen scowl and insult the audience in her tough Scouse accent. She is hilarious, and she is here four nights a week. Your beer is warm by the time your friend brings it from the bar. Cheers and laughter, bodies and lights. *I am what I am.* There is nowhere like this – this boisterous Vauxhall pub that was raided by police seeking poppers in 1986.

The first raid came just days after a newspaper article decrying the legal sale of poppers inside. The police tore in, made arrests and seized bottles of poppers from behind the bar. Many more officers came on the second raid, some with surgical gloves this time. "The police officer next to me was wearing rubber gloves and I said to my other half, 'We haven't all got AIDS'," recalled Ken Comish. After he spoke out, he was arrested on suspicion of being drunk in a pub. Prosecutions followed from these raids, but the process was long, delayed, troubled.

From the drag queen's frock to the police gloves and the judge's wig, the whole production was a big show and dance.

There is some important set dressing for this show at the Royal Vauxhall Tavern, which was built in 1860 and since the 1970s has been central to London's queer scene. The first piece of dressing was the police attitude towards men who had sex with each other. Britain's police forces have a dark history of persecuting them. By the mid-80s this had been going on for decades – in fact, after the partial decriminalisation of sex acts between men in 1967, police actions only increased. Using other laws to persecute gay men, police trapped them in public toilets and stormed into their pubs. When AIDS was associated with gay sex, the police had even more excuses. Gay sex was seen a matter of public health; pubs as a vector of infection. In 1984 the Report of the Metropolitan Police Commissioner proposed tolerating only one gay pub per district.[1]

The second piece of the set dressing was the perception that poppers were a lethal substance on a par with heroin. On June 22nd, 1986, an article in the *Sunday Mirror* linked poppers to the high-profile death of a young woman called Olivia Channon. She was the daughter of the Secretary of Trade and a member of the wealthy Guinness family. She died aged twenty-two after taking too many drugs, including heroin and alcohol. Olivia mixed with wealthy socialites who could get anything and everything they wanted. The night of her death was a party in a fellow student's room at Christ Church College.[2]

Although there is no reporting that poppers were present at the fatal party, eleven days after she died a reporter for the *Sunday Mirror* saw poppers "being sold at Olivia's favourite nightclub, The Coven" in Oxford. The journalist made a very elastic connection of the type that is beloved of the British tabloids. "Sex drug for sale" said the resulting headline, beneath the words "Students defy lesson of Olivia's death". You'd hope that a journalist would know that if there is a lesson to learn from Olivia's death, it is not to take too much heroin. But the story, linking a glamorous dead heiress with a sex drug, was too good not to print – even if the link was only a dotted line. Tabloid reporters love doing this, performing a role that is part magician, part judge. They conjure the facts into something just solid enough to knock down with a hammer. The result in this case was a story in a widely read newspaper that implied poppers were lethal.

The third thing setting the stage for the raid was the horror of AIDS, an epidemic and a crisis by 1986. Many people were ignorant that it was caused by HIV, and exactly how this virus was transmitted. The volunteers at Switchboard encountered this ignorance and prejudice directly when they needed their phone lines fixed. "BT engineers would not come into the phone room at Switchboard because they thought they'd get AIDS," said Lisa Power, one of the volunteers at the time, on *The Log Books* podcast. "They were literally afraid that they would get AIDS by working on the phone lines outside of our building, which was so ridiculous we thought it wasn't true."[3]

The fears connecting gays, their hedonism, disease and death were extreme. On December 7th, 1986, the *Sunday Telegraph* ran a story with the headline, "Poppers, the new danger drug in the pub, as easy to buy as crisps". The drug was declared a "deadly craze" (not true) that was "sweeping through Britain's teenagers" (unverified). This second claim relied on a story related to the reporters by a man who was about to enter the Royal Vauxhall Tavern when he was asked by two teens to buy them some poppers.

As well as reporting the sale of poppers at the RVT, the journalists also found them on sale at the Britannia pub in Bethnal Green and Bromptons in Earl's Court. The mention of these three pubs combined with later police actions means it is almost certain that the police read this article in the *Sunday Telegraph*. The expert quoted in the story was Patrick Toseland, a toxicologist at Guy's Hospital, who analysed the poppers bought by the reporters and found a mixture of alkyl nitrites, mostly amyl nitrite (he also appears later in this story). "In my opinion, excessive use by inhalation is much more dangerous than a larger quantity swallowed," he told the journalists, although this opinion is surely wrong. The *Telegraph* story ends with the ultimate kicker: death. There is a widespread fear, it claims, that sniffing amyl nitrite can make "users more vulnerable to the killer AIDS virus".

Fear of gay men, fear of death, fear of rampant teenagers, fear of AIDS... the stage was set for a big show. The curtains went up on the night of Wednesday, December 17th, 1986.

Imagine the police officers, specifically their bodies, in the moments just before the raid itself. There is the face of a young man, seriously attending to the careful plan spoken by his superior. There are his hands and his arms, pulling on his shirt, his jacket, his helmet. Imagine this young man's counterpart, inside the pub, specifically his body, in jeans and a denim jacket, hugging a friend hello, or resting his head on his lover's shoulder, hand in the back pocket. Eyes front, they are watching the queen on the stage, ripping through her gags, their mouths opening with laughter. Imagine the police officer's body colliding into the punters' bodies. His is pushing theirs back – what, in this moment, does the future look like?

Seven police officers stormed into the RVT with a search warrant. They seized poppers from behind the bar and arrested Breda and Pat McConnon, the landlady and landlord, and three staff. Being held in a cell was a particular stress for Breda, who suffered claustrophobia and needed medical attention. A doctor gave her a Valium to take when she got home. "I'm bloody taking it now!" she said.[4]

This raid was merely an opening act. The year turned over into January 1987, a crucial month in the HIV/ AIDS epidemic. The government had printed twenty-three million copies of a leaflet, one for every household in the country, ready for mailing. The leaflet would explain candidly how HIV was transmitted, how condoms would protect sex partners from it, and where people could find more information. Writing in *Capital Gay* that month, Tony Whitehead said that the leaflet "certainly goes a lot further than traditional Tory voters would wish and will unleash a storm of protest. January will be another busy month for AIDS in the media."[5] He braced the gay community for further attacks.

But people were still going out, of course. Not even an epidemic or the threat of attack could keep everyone at home. The tabloids were screaming "gay plague!" in an effort to ratchet up hostility between people, but the RVT thumped on like an enduring human heart, filled with drag and cabaret acts, dancing, drinking, friends, lovers, hooking up. The pub was also a place that people retreated to after losing someone to an AIDS-related illness. Mostly it was a place of joy and freedom. On January 23rd, the early show was John Thomas and the Cockettes. The late show was a very popular drag queen, Lily Savage. She was on stage when the police burst in.[6]

Imagine that young officer again, this time in a van outside the target location, snapping on the same gloves that surgeons use when they cut into people's bodies. There were thirty-five officers this time, and they pushed themselves into the pub. Savage says she remembers telling the crowd to riot, and she was one of the people taken to the police station that night.

Somebody phoned Switchboard at 2am on the 24th to report the raid, including the fact that some officers were wearing "rubber gloves". The Switchboard volunteer wrote in the log book: "No apparent 'reason' for raid. Several arrests." Two more people had phoned by 3am, and another call came through at 4.40am to report that twelve people had been arrested, most released.[7] The landlord Pat McConnon was among those arrested, again, along with his bar staff, on suspicion of breaking fire safety regulations. Punters were arrested for being drunk. "[I'd had] two pints," said Ken Comish in a BBC documentary, "I was just on my third."[8]

Comish later claimed that the police harmed him that night. At the time of his arrest he was recovering from an operation to remove some cartilage in his knee. In the station, the police surgeon peeled back Comish's dressing and "sent him away with blood pouring down his leg", according to stories in *Capital Gay* in 1988.[9] Comish had turned to the newspaper to appeal for witnesses to support his action against the police for unlawful detention, unlawful imprisonment and assault.

Comish's mistreatment at the hands of the police is doubly insulting given officers' apparent care to protect themselves. It is the gloves that stick in the mind. The police were not searching people or doing anything medical. They may have had to touch people as they seized control of the pub, but there seemed no sensible reason for the gloves except the fear of HIV transmission. Nurses, doctors and patients knew that HIV could not be transmitted through casual contact; it was not until Diana, the Princess of Wales, shook the hand of a person living with AIDS that finally made most people understand this fact about the virus. But that historic handshake wouldn't happen until April that year. At the time of their raid on the RVT, the police seemed to think they could catch HIV by touch. So some people in the pub thought the gloves were a symbol of police ignorance about how HIV is transmitted. Others deemed it an insult towards a group of people the police deemed too loathsome to touch.

Exactly what were the police officers doing? They might say they were enforcing the law. But if they wanted to protect people from harmful substances, they should have removed the cigarette machine. If they wanted to stop people from being drunk, they should have gone to other types of pub too. Enforcement of actual laws is not even the half of it. Really they were showing off the fact that they had the authority and power to step into a place and stop whatever was happening. And not just any place – the few spaces where lesbians, gay people and other sexual and gender minorities could meet. Police also raided Stallions, a Sunday afternoon tea dance for queer people held in a back street off Tottenham Court Road. Stallions did not even serve alcohol. It is almost impossible to conclude anything about these linked police actions other than that they wanted to intimidate people. And they had tacit approval from government.

They even had allyship from abroad. Police officers in the USA were also wearing gloves in the presence of gay men. Specifically, they arrived at protests against their government's mishandling of AIDS with their hands covered. In response, activists began to wear yellow kitchen gloves, most notably on a demonstration outside the Supreme Court in Washington DC in October 1987. Michael Lynch got fellow activists to sign his glove and he turned it into a piece of art.[10]

In Britain, the prime minister did not want to touch the issue. But she did like to say that the whole thing of AIDS was a matter of morality. In defending the chief constable of Greater Manchester who had blamed gays for AIDS, Margaret Thatcher told parliament on January 29th: "Some people, whether from the Church or elsewhere, had spoken out to the effect that morals do matter in AIDS and that, while Governments cannot prevent people from getting AIDS, people themselves, by their own conduct, can do so."

Thatcher overlooked Christians like Dudley Cave, a Switchboard volunteer, and those who set up the Mildmay Mission Hospital in Shoreditch, Europe's first dedicated HIV hospice. Unlike Thatcher, they were responding compassionately to people with HIV, not just condemning them. But the Conservative government was dogged in its disdain for people with HIV and, by association, all gay people. On February 2nd, a junior minister at the Home Office, Douglas Hogg, published a written answer to a question in parliament, explaining why the police had worn gloves at the RVT. His note said they were "to protect officers from the risk of infection by hepatitis B or AIDS as a result of accidental injury from any drugs paraphernalia which might have been found on individuals searched during the operation". (He also admitted that although one of the stated reasons for the raid was to investigate drunkenness, no such complaints had been made by Vauxhall residents.)[11]

On the same day that Hogg made his statement, police moved in on an address in Rochester, Kent. Here they seized amyl nitrite and other chemicals said to be worth £40,000. Poppers were not illegal, nor was their manufacture or their sale. So the charges, when they eventually came, had to describe amyl nitrite as a poison, and the defendants as snakes. The landlord of the RVT, Pat McConnon, barman Paul Blackburn, plus those associated with the Rochester address, John "Jim" Breen, Paul Strain and Kevin Quarmby, were charged with conspiracy to administer a noxious substance with intent to injure, under Section 24 of the Offences Against the Person Act from 1861.

In the same month, one of the Cockettes, the group that had been playing on the night of the second raid, was hit by a Ford Escort. Melanie Sharp had been loading the car ready for a gig in Hammersmith when the passing vehicle struck her. "She flew across the pavement," bandmate John Thomas told *Capital Gay*.[12] Meanwhile, the phone lines at Switchboard were overloading due to the surge in calls from people who had seen the number on the government HIV/AIDS leaflet – these calls used the faulty lines that had been avoided by BT. On February 22nd, Andy Warhol died in New York. It was not a good start to the year.

The BBC took an interest in the raids at the RVT. Television producers were more interested in police in gloves than poppers, though. So they worked on reconstructing the second raid for an episode of *Heart of the Matter*, a documentary series examining social and religious affairs. At the start of the programme, Lily Savage takes to the stage for the reconstruction quipping: "Some queens get *EastEnders*. What do I get? Bloody religious programme, half past ten on a Sunday night, for god's sake."

The documentary is essentially a collection of interviews extracted by the sharp questioning of Helena Kennedy. She speaks to a couple of lords, an erudite prof, a Victorian Tory MP, and a couple of punters including Ken Comish quoted at the top of this chapter. But it is her conversation with Mike Farbrother, the man selected by the police force to front its defence, that is most telling. "The purpose of the raid was to detect drunkenness on the premises," he says, deadpan. Kennedy asks why the police failed to announce that intention on the mic they seized, to which Farbrother responds with a truth universally acknowledged: "One can never be sure that drunkenness is going to take place in one particular individual at a particular time."

He repeated the Home Office minister's earlier claim that the gloves protected the police from infection. "We've had a number of cases of police officers who've actually contracted hepatitis B as a result of actually having pricked their fingers on needles in people's pockets," Farbrother said, seeming to believe that a surgical glove can block a sharp prick, which it cannot. The editor of the programme cuts from Farbrother to one of his colleagues, an anonymous gay officer shown only in silhouette, who says, "I don't know why they give us gloves because they don't protect you in any way from a needle or syringe or even a piece of glass... It's a gross form of insult."

When Farbrother told Kennedy that the gloves were used for the purposes of a drugs search, she replied that no one was searched. "I can't confirm or deny that," he said. The past is shaped by what is said in the present. He sat through the interview, backed by books about public order, in a glistening white shirt trimmed on the shoulders with his epaulettes and rank slides. His face is flat, even when he knows he is saying nonsense. It's quite the performance.

Geoffrey Dickens puts on a decent show too – but the man was known for this. Dickens was a northern working-class Conservative Member of Parliament with a booming voice full of opinions. He had one for everything, including dangerous teddy bears (ban them) and hanging (bring it back).[13] Under the scrutiny of Kennedy, in the *Heart of the Matter* broadcast on March 8th, 1987, Dickens revealed what seemed to be on the minds of his constituents, and perhaps even the police who had raided the RVT.

There are gay and lesbian clubs all over the place, he said, almost embodying a Spartacus guide to London for a moment. "We find they have regular meeting places, we find they have certain pubs which they frequent and they entice and corrupt and bring others into their net... An unnatural net, in a sense." He suggested that the partial decriminalisation of homosexuality in 1967 ought to be rethought, perhaps to make it harder for men to have sex with each other: "Sometimes we have to interfere in civil liberties to do what is right."

Kennedy prodded at this complex character, a man who looks like a teddy bear with pink cheeks. She was especially interested in his understanding of liberty. And she was particularly good at this, with every contributor – but that is because she is a human rights barrister. Although Kennedy was credited as the film's "reporter", off screen she had already spent more than a decade at the bar. She had worked on some of the most important cases to do with women's rights, and had even defended the men entrapped by police in public toilets when seeking sex with other men. As a reporter, she gives a gripping performance. No wonder the programme ended up focusing less on specific raids and more on the principles of civil liberty.

Kennedy's contributors also hit on a debate about the family, and how they thought this idea was threatened at the time by people in same-sex relationships. "The tragedy of such people is that they cannot enjoy family life and they cannot have children," said Frank Pakenham, also known as the Earl of Longford, in the House of Lords, around this time.[14] This is an enduring idea, used to clamp down on sexual freedom. As Dickens declares in his interview with Kennedy, "the family life in this country is eroding for all sorts of reasons and one of the components may well be the liberalisation of sexual attitudes". He is careful not to say that his idea of a family is eroding because too many people are having same-sex pleasure, but that is clearly what he means. He would find an ally in the mother who contributed to an episode of *The London Programme* from April 1987, about why she did not want homosexuality to be promoted to her son. "I want him to be normal," she says, straight-faced, "to have children of his own."[15]

These traditionalists are all interested in the future – but it seems the only legitimate future is the one arrived at through the transmission of genetic material down the generations, within mixed-sex relationships. Their claims of course gained more power as the numbers of HIV infections and AIDS deaths rose. Dickens stood for mainstream Conservative Party family values when he put the blame for this illness not with a virus but with a group of people doing certain sex acts. "I'm afraid this sort of behaviour is totally unacceptable," he said on national television. "You're putting your nation at risk by your behaviour, we're not gonna have this in the future, and that's why [we should say] we're now legislating again to make it once again a crime to commit these sorts of offences."

From March to September 1987, the defendants connected to the RVT and the apparent manufacture of poppers in Kent were in and out of court. Pat McConnon was charged with permitting drunkenness in his pub in one court appearance. The case was thrown out on another date, because the police had failed to submit evidence. All the police had wanted was to intimidate landlords like McConnon and to show lawmakers like Hogg and Dickens that they were ready to close down gay pubs if the time came. In April, the intimidation continued. Police officers walked into three gay pubs across London to check their licenses.

Two of the three pubs were the Britannia in Bethnal Green and Bromptons in Earl's Court, which had both been named in the *Sunday Telegraph* story as places where poppers were on sale. "The local police are very friendly. We think these weren't local because if they were they would know about our hours," said Nicky Amin from the Britannia pub, quoted in *Capital Gay*.[16] "It's very weird. I don't know what they are trying to do."

The poppers case must have seemed serious. Many pubs stopped selling poppers as a precaution, as they watched the RVT case travel through the court system. It was set back and back, though. First it was delayed so that the police and prosecutors could assemble more medical and scientific reports on the substances seized. They tried to delay it again but could not produce the required amount of evidence for that. In May 1987, a judge called for poppers to be banned after he heard a case of a young man from Bromley who both sniffed poppers and stabbed a fourteen-year-old girl. Judge John Hazan QC told the court that poppers caused hallucinations and intensified feelings, and also wrote to the Home Office to plead for their prohibition. It is a strange and sad story, churned up by the report in the *Sun* newspaper on May 30th: "A judge yesterday called for a ban on a sex potion which turned a well-behaved teenager into a crazed knifeman."

The *News on Sunday*, a new left-wing paper that went bankrupt after six weeks, took up the story too: "The sex thrill that can kill" was the headline on June 7th. Using the Bromley case as a peg, one of the *News on Sunday* reporters put the judge's claims to the manager of a sex shop in Soho selling poppers. "He was chased down the street and told not to return," according to the story. The piece also quotes Alan Billington, an anti-drugs campaigner who claimed that two young people per week killed themselves after sniffing poppers or other solvents. "The figures don't account for people who did crazy things after sniffing poppers," he said, "kids who jumped out of windows or walked under buses while they were high... In many cases, they make kids so high they don't know what they are doing." You might wonder what Billington himself was sniffing.

In July the RVT/Kent poppers case was delayed for more scientific tests, and finally in September a hearing date was set for December. The prosecution built its case on the possible harmful effects of amyl nitrite, pulling in three expert witnesses with claims to make against the substance. First up: Ronald Wood, a professor of environmental medicine at New York University. Wood told the court that inhaling poppers deeply could lead to methemoglobinemia (starving vital organs of oxygen), but admitted that no deaths had occurred from this. Next to testify was Guy Newell, a doctor of medicine at Tulane University, who had been publishing work in the USA making the correlation between using poppers and developing Kaposi's sarcoma. According to the report of this hearing in *Capital Gay* on December 18th,[17] under cross examination Newell "confessed that his theories had been dismissed by AIDS authorities all over the world". The third expert was a local: Patrick Toseland from Guy's Hospital in London – the toxicologist who had been quoted in the *Sunday Telegraph* article that may have inspired the raid in the first place.

One of the defence barristers argued that amyl nitrite was lawful, but the trying of the defendants for supplying a "noxious substance" meant that anyone supplying alcohol and tobacco also ought to be tried for the same. Another defence barrister dared to pose a reason for the prosecution to want poppers to be made illegal. They "may be undesirable in certain quarters because they encourage promiscuity in the gay community," he said. When the judge was told how some people like to sniff amyl nitrite which can smell like a locker room, he said, "A locker room? Like one might find in a golf club?"

From one theatre of the establishment to another: the judge committed the case to a full trial at the Old Bailey, London's central criminal court. At that stage, a year after the raid at the RVT, it seemed like the defendants would have to wait another year for their day in court. While they waited, the RVT was raided again. Police marched in at 22:15 on Sunday, June 5th, 1988, during a show that involved screening a mix of films such as *Whatever Happened to Baby Jane*.[18] The compere of the night was Lily Savage (again), who had to scramble to stop the film when the police arrived. The charge this time was that the McConnons, the landlords, didn't have a licence to play videos.

After obtaining a video licence, the McConnons resumed their wait for the poppers trial. It took some time: the raid had happened in December 1986, and it was not until March 1989 that the trial began. Over a few days of legal argument, the judge became so unimpressed by the prosecution that the whole show collapsed.[19] The judge ruled that the prosecution had failed to make a case that the defendants had conspired to cause people to take a noxious substance, so he ordered the jury to return a verdict of not guilty. The five defendants walked free. They were able to go back to their lives running a pub and distributing poppers. "It was just two years of worry, with all this hanging over me," said Breen, quoted in *Capital Gay*, which had followed the case diligently for more than two years.

In 2014, a person dressed up as a police officer to make another performance in the RVT. Jade Pollard-Crowe strutted onto the stage wearing a police uniform, headscarf and rubber gloves.[20] Mixing striptease, parody and the smooth sound of "Let's Groove" by Earth, Wind and Fire, Pollard-Crowe re-enacted the police raid from 1987 and received laughter and applause. The performance was not only a piece of fun. "As both a queer lesbian and a Black body," Pollard-Crowe told me, "impersonating a police officer was a complex and convoluted act." In mimicking police brutality towards Black bodies and those in the QUILTBAG, it referenced the poppers raid, the police's long-established practice of racial profiling, and the imposition of white power on people of colour. That the show managed to elicit laughs while also unpicking these awful realities makes it a queer performance. The rubber gloves raid had become a legend, ready to be re-performed by an artist with something to say, and written about here as an excuse for saying something about the worlds we build for our bodies to live in.

Whether the year is 2014 or 3014, we cannot look back on those raids and not think about the future they pre-dated. Alongside the image of police officers in surgical gloves storming into a gay pub we can place the surreal future that actually came to be: that of police officers clipping rainbow ribbons to their uniforms and dancing in the middle of a Pride parade. That is where we are now. Many forces even have vans featuring a rainbow version of the police badge and the slogan "Police with Pride". It is dizzying to zip back and forth between the images of police at Pride today and at the Royal Vauxhall Tavern in 1986 and 1987.

The raids show what happens when groups of people clash over their different ideas of the future. Everyone is on a stage, performing a future they want. Traditionalists talk up their idea of the family, and down the idea of an alternative, or queerness. Lawyers act out in court the facts that they want to become accepted truth. Police officers seek to secure their place in the future by a show of force today. Drag queens and other performers wear what they want and speak their minds, embodying the freer future they want for us all. Punters laugh, drink and dance late – stretching tonight into tomorrow. And people who want a sexual moment to go a little deeper, to last a little longer, find that their poppers are in police custody.

The poppers seized by police in December 1986 and February 1987 were destined mainly to be bought by gay men. If they had not been taken away, these poppers would have been used to deepen these men's intimate connections, to make them feel more joy as they danced together, even intensified their orgasms. They could have even broken free of their point-of-sale placement and marketing categories, landing under the nostrils of women, or trans, non-binary, straight people, improving all manner of intimate connections. In fact, sniffing poppers can make you feel like the moment you are living in is better. If you're having sex, it can feel more pleasurable. If you have a good connection with the partner, it can feel even deeper. The world falls away. That present, *better* moment is essentially the future you hope for – why can't it always be like this?

A better future is the thing we expect to see imagined by musicians, dancers, artists, actors, drag queens – they can all show us an alternative to the present. The reason why queer performance is such a big part of queer culture is because it creates a better world to inhabit, just for a moment. The star on the stage dares to wear the body/clothing combinations that traditionalists might object to, or that *Grazia* magazine might disdain. They can talk (or sing) about things that get only rare mentions in the office or on television talk shows. They can embody themselves as they wish. They can invert the power dynamics that usually hold them down, just as Pollard-Crowe parodied the gloved policemen.

Good queer performers push their audiences forward into the future they desire. A good performance is utopia for a moment.

In the Royal Vauxhall Tavern, all of these potential utopias were willed away when the police stormed in. Performances interrupted, orgasms foregone, connections broken – the police brought their alternative performance. The police did not just want to stop what was happening; they wanted to make their own utopia for a moment. They pulled on their costumes and they put themselves to work on embodying authority, power, intimidation. As individual officers, people with homes and hobbies, they had been moved by some newspaper stories about a deadly sex craze and by others that spoke of a horrible illness killing men who had sex with each other. They heard the words of politicians who spoke about preserving families and protecting children. As individuals they may even have wanted no more gay or queer people. As an organised group of individuals each wanting to belong to something bigger than they were, police officers were grabbed by the idea of cutting the number of queer venues. All we have is the records of their group performance: the way they stopped gay and queer people. They arrested our futures, at least for a night or two.

The story of these raids is a story from the past, but it is about how we live in the present, creating a future. In every moment we are performing, making choices about the future we want to build for ourselves and others. We can be inspired by other people who are better than us at articulating a future. But it is not some distant, formless thing. How we are living now is always creating a future, whether or not we like it. Whether or not we are trying, we are performing a future. As a genderqueer dancer stretches the limbs they have, they bring us into their utopia for a moment.

Until I had sex I hadn't realised that many gay men divide their bodies into "being" either a top or a bottom.

I was twenty-nine, discovering that my body was what they call versatile.

6. A Guilty Pleasure

Mother Superior Mary Regina peers into a bag that one of her sisters has found in a school bathroom. She pulls out a small glass bottle, reads the word "Rush" from the label, and says, "It must be for people in a hurry." Of course she takes a whiff of the poppers, and within seconds the nun's body is flushed with the holy spirit. "Ooooh, is it hot in here?" she asks her audience, who are already laughing. As her rush builds and she sniffs again, the scene gets even more ridiculous. The other sisters appear, and they start to tap dance and sing a song called "Tackle That Temptation with a Time Step".

It's always funny to watch a nun experience a little pleasure. It is a physical joke as old as a face full of cream pie – and funny for the same reason. Dignity is lost. Respectability, inverted. Propriety, interrupted. The mother superior sniffing poppers is the climax to act one of the musical *Nunsense*. The scene requires some excellent face work from the main performer, with her eyes crossed and mouth ajar in an exaggerated high. Played well, the joke is a riot and the audience returns after the interval jeered up and wanting more.

The portrayal of poppers in *Nunsense* places pleasure at the service of humour. In fact, if you take a trip through the many representations of poppers in Western culture in the English language, you will see that pleasure is never primary and is often not included at all. Just like a lot of sex education, pleasure is the bottom priority after all the talk about mechanics, pregnancy and disease. Things like sex toys and poppers are excluded from sex education even though they are aids to pleasure, except perhaps where they are mentioned as a warning. Poppers are linked to shame and death always before they are linked to pleasure, which is intriguing given that pleasure is the number one reason they are used. If your eyes and ears are open for poppers, you'll have your own cultural references rather than relying on the ones in this chapter. And they are almost certainly going to place poppers only as a guilty pleasure.

That is, at least, a successful storytelling device. Since its first performance in 1985, *Nunsense* has become one of the most successful off-Broadway musicals in history. It is a global franchise, with more than five thousand productions in many countries, eight sequels, merchandise for sale and even a line of nun's habits available for rent via FedEx. This means that hundreds of performers on different nights in different theatres have pulled on a habit, sniffed poppers and made thousands of people laugh. Fake nuns with fake rushes have aroused real joy all around the world.

Nunsense is probably not the first piece of entertainment to play poppers for laughs. But its appearance in 1985 certainly coincided with the start of a trend of this. As Sam Goggin sat down in New York to write the scene where a nun sniffs from a bottle of Rush, another artist on the other side of the USA was sketching out a comic strip.

It started as a side gig. Jerry Mills was simply dreaming up a memorable set of scenarios and realistic caricatures to mock. Billy is a blonde, white himbo whose life revolves around partying and fucking. His best friend Yves is also white and hunky, but a little more plain-faced and boring. Their pairing gave Mills the license to explore the vanity of the gay male world in West Hollywood, where the strip was set. The less frequent character André, a cool Black queen, adds wisdom. And the humour comes from Buster, the crab louse who lives in Billy's pubic hair. The boys trip through bars and beaches, and Buster gets to hang out with other crabs every time Billy hooks up.

In one early strip, Yves and Billy are in a bar but Yves is not enjoying the music. Billy tries to loosen him up by saying, "Here, Yves! Have a hit of poppers! Sniff!" But Yves isn't having it. "No thanks!" he says. "And where's your shirt?" But Billy is now cross-eyed, his head spinning, his tongue hanging, his dick hard and going SPROING. A thought bubble arises from Yves: "Disgusting!"

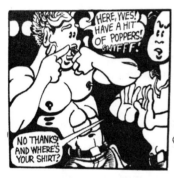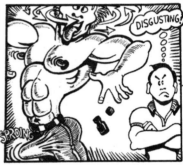

This single panel portraying the difference between Billy's overactive dick and Yves's judgements set the tone for the strip that was named *Poppers*. Mill's creation started to appear in the adult magazine *In Touch for Men* in the early 1980s. He was working in the magazine's subscriptions department but the editor John Calendo gave his comic a place on the page. Mills' stories of haircuts and sex, love and beaches, muscles and crabs became popular. *Poppers* ran for years and even gained syndication abroad. In France it appeared in *Gai Pied*, the magazine that was named by Michel Foucault, the philosopher of sex and other things.

Mills' *Poppers* is filled with humour, often visual gags drawn by the hand of a very skilled cartoonist. There is a real sense of comic timing and pacing between the panels.

When Yves calls Billy a "sexual compulsive", Billy denies it. Meanwhile... his eyes are checking out another guy and his thought bubble is saying, "Gee, he's cute".

The stories poke fun at their characters. Yves addresses his lack of social confidence by privately reading a book about being assertive. Billy gets addicted to his VCR. Billy teaches Yves how to wash spinach in the shower. The boys have to decide between bars with names like Standaround, Man-load, Baskets and Zero's. Their adventures often revolve around the fun of double lives. In one strip, Billy and Yves drag up for Halloween and flirt with some dudes in a country bar who complain about all the local faggots. Our boys decide to teach these dudes a lesson, so they take them to a motel and reveal their true bodies. The dudes, still keen, say "Sure! What the hell!" and Billy and Yves collapse in shock.

Naturally for a piece of work named after poppers, the strip is as sexy as it is funny. Although the characters are just cartoons, they are beautiful – especially their bodies, in the style of what was considered most attractive in this time and place. Mills draws bulging crotches, curvy bums and perfect muscles. In one tantalising scene, Billy and Yves end up in a motel orgy with some marines, sniffing poppers on the bed. (Buster meets his marine equivalents, who spend their time marching back and forth among their owners' pubes.)

Poppers is designed to make the reader laugh, and especially to feel implicated in its satire of the gay male culture in West Hollywood in the early 1980s. The world of *Poppers* is full of sex, or at least the pursuit of it, and the vanities and insecurities of gay men. Mills clearly based the characters, bodies and locations on his own observations – just like Goggin, the creator of *Nunsense*. Goggin based his musical on five nuns who taught him at Catholic school in Michigan. "We never wanted to get into anything political or anything like that because we weren't about that," he said in an interview in 2015. "I think there's a place for shows like that. But our idea was just to make you laugh."[1]

Nunsense started as a cabaret show in Greenwich Village in New York City, booked for four weekends. This first run ended up lasting for thirty-eight weeks. Popular demand led Goggin to flesh out his characters and expand the cabaret into a full musical. "People kept saying, 'We want to know more about the real characters and their stories', and that's really what propelled it," he said. "We wanted to find out who these people were."

The combination of nuns and the queer neighbourhood that was Greenwich Village in the 1980s meant that poppers were an inevitable gag. Goggin must have known that his audience would know all about poppers, just as Mills' audience knew all about gay vanity. Both creators used poppers in their most famous works for jokes, but with something more too. The use of poppers is in fact an in-joke, a marker for audience members from a specific community with a specific set of experiences.

Creators of non-fiction have played poppers for laughs too. On March 6th, 1989, the *Sun* newspaper published a story featuring poppers, a nightclub and a lion.[2] It is a classic in the genre of tabloid titillation, and it was written by a journalist called Neil Wallis. By the story's own claim, the tale is "bizarre and outrageous", but the style of the piece suggests it was written more for humour than anything else. "The night gays fled from love-drug lion" is the headline on the double-page spread, which is also splashed with the words "Inside secrets of the Hippodrome".

That strapline refers to *The Hippodrome Show*, in which scenes from the London nightclub were broadcast on ITV on Wednesday nights to ten million viewers. The Hippodrome was owned by Peter Stringfellow, who had a chain of famous clubs associated with celebrities, glamour and sleaze. On one of the Hippodrome's gay nights, which was to be featured in an episode of the television show, the organisers decided to programme what Wallis's story called "a perfect stunt for the outrageous gay night – a cowardly lion!" The lion, whose name was Queen Bluey, was not necessarily cowardly by nature. She was tranquilised so that the patrons in the club could pet her. But the story hinges on the claim that the lion was affected by all the poppers vapour in the air. "As soon as the lion got one whiff of that it went berserk," according to the club's former press officer, Paul Kassell, who is quoted in the story. "I've never seen anything so 'high' in all my life."

The witness went on to claim that Queen Bluey's eyes were popping out of her head, she was gasping for breath, whining and growling. She ran off the stage and tore around the club. "We ended up with hundreds of squealing gays running over each other in every direction, stabbing each other with their false nails in their panic," said Kassell. The double-page spread featured a main photograph of the lion after she had been caught in a net, just before being carried away. There are also little portraits of some of the club's clients. One tattooed reveller was labelled as "BIZARRE" and two genderqueer people who were photographed kissing were labelled as "ODD COUPLE".

There is a lot going on in this story. The snooty language about queer people was common in the printed press in the 1980s, and remains a dark stain on the UK's media history. Much has been written about that, but what may not have been covered previously is the portrayal of poppers. Who knows if the lioness was really responding to poppers, rather than the fact that as she came up from a hit of tranquilizer she found herself in a nightclub surrounded by sweaty humans. Who knows if she really galloped around the club as reported in the story. Wallis's story quotes only one source, this guy Kassell, a press officer no less. Who knows if the "squealing gays" really stabbed each other with their false nails. The thing about news stories like this one, in tabloids like the *Sun*, is that they often stretch the truth or make things up. So really all we can know here is that Wallis and his editors saw this story as newsworthy because of its combination of gays, poppers and a lion.

Wallis's story is designed to surprise and amuse the reader. (That is the charitable interpretation; the story may also have wanted to engender hostility towards queer people and some of their culture.) As with Goggin's musical and Mills' comic, in the lion story there is something funny about poppers.

Writing about poppers can also be funny when it covers certain individuals indulging in a sniff. On November 23rd, 2007, several writers for different news organisations reported claims that Kate Moss, the model, had sniffed poppers at a friend's birthday party. The story seems to have come from the night's DJ, Elliot Eastwick, who told Stewart Maclean at the *Mirror*, "Kate pulled some poppers out of her handbag and started snorting them in really heavily. It went straight to her head. You could see her loll as it took effect." The fact that a person sniffed poppers – that is the story. It appeared with the same angle on many different websites, including those of *Marie Claire* and even *China Daily*, the newspaper owned by the publicity department of the Chinese Communist Party.

A year later it was the turn of Gordon Ramsay, a celebrity chef. No fewer than four reporters for the *Daily Mail* and *Mail Online* covered the story on November 24th, 2008, that Ramsay was having an affair that involved sniffing poppers.[3] He had been meeting a person who the journalists describe as a "professional mistress" in a hotel. Shopping before one of her meetings with Ramsay, the woman bought two bottles of white wine, a bag of crisps and three bottles of Rave and Rush poppers.

In December 2019, singers Sam Smith and Nicole Scherzinger were being observed with poppers too. A person spotted them sniffing in a club in Soho in London, and soon posted about it online. The news was covered in mainstream newspapers like the *Sun* and in LGBTQ+ specialist media like *PinkNews*, which described the scene as a "moment of religious significance".[4] In April 2020, when Smith was pressed into talking more about that night, they answered, "I can completely confirm – I love poppers... I've been ashamed to say that, but I have so much fun when I do poppers."[5]

No one really needs to know that this celebrity was sniffing poppers. But anyway, the *PinkNews* story is doing more than just sharing gossip. The full headline is "Ally of the year Nicole Scherzinger 'sniffed poppers' at a gay bar with Sam Smith and we have no legal choice but to stan". The story creates a sense of community with its readers by asserting the "religious experience" of sniffing poppers as a gay activity. The involvement of Scherzinger, who is not gay, makes her an ally to gay people like Smith. Every detail that is given weight in the story re-performs the category of "gay". Every detail confirms that people who are already connected to gay life are involved in this, and they are doing good things. Every detail makes the story clickable and shareable by gay people. It's the type of story that performs well for online publishers like *PinkNews*: it re-affirms a group identity.

There are other online news stories about poppers and famous people, specifically those that come from tell-all memoirs. The books themselves are not enough, it seems; they are sliced up by online writers who pull out specific passages and turn them into fresh stories. One such book is that of Mimi Alford, who was a mistress of John F. Kennedy during his presidency. In her memoir she recalls a party at the desert ranch of the singer Bing Crosby, which she attended along with Kennedy. "I was sitting next to him in the living room when a handful of yellow capsules – most likely amyl nitrate [sic], commonly known as poppers – was offered up by one of the guests," Alford writes. "The president asked me if I wanted to try the drug, which stimulated the heart but also purportedly enhanced sex. I said no, but he just went ahead and popped the capsule and held it under my nose."

This story is one of the main ones included in a brief write-up of the memoir by the *New York Post* website.[6] It details more of Alford and Kennedy's sex life, describing it as varied and fun, and involving lots of baths. But the specific notion of a president on poppers is the most detailed section of the story.

Another gossipy news site, *Page Six*, posted an article in July 2020 about the artist Brigid Berlin, who worked and socialised with Andy Warhol. When she inherited $150,000 from a pal of her dad's, she spent it on Cartier jewellery, "a hundred cold lobsters from Seville... [and] I also ordered like a hundred boxes of poppers."[7]

Alford and Berlin lived in close proximity to famous men whose sex lives were of deep interest to the world in the twentieth century. Their stories about poppers are short and hardly substantial, but the fact that they are recorded and bounced again by online news articles indicates something of a cultural obsession. These stories are about luxury and decadence – poppers, like the lobsters bought by Berlin, are a form of pleasure that others would seek, if they could, or if they dared. Pleasure also pulses between the lines in the tabloids and news sites covering celebrities using poppers. Part of the titillation around, say, Gordon Ramsay's alleged affair is the revelation that it involved him seeking pleasure with poppers. Sam Smith at least declared that they love poppers, which perhaps took the sting out of the tabloid-style exposure that they were sniffing them on a night out.

All these writers, whether they are inventing the comedic

exploits of nuns or himbos, or covering the revelations of real people who sniff, are doing something strange with how we think about pleasure. They may be writing for laughs or gossip, but they are also always building a distance between our bodies and the pleasures we can enjoy in them. Even the story of Smith declaring their love of poppers is framed as the singer "finally addressing the rumours". That story is not about Smith's pleasure, despite their own words to that effect, but rather about the fact of a revelation. The story is also used to re-affirm the category "gay", in a celebration targeted at the idea of a gay community. The story is even written from the perspective of a "we". When we talk of poppers, it seems we have to make them anything other than just a simple pleasure.

Often, especially in fiction, pleasure is the very opposite of how poppers are portrayed. Poppers are seen to kill characters, or at least be near when death appears. This only adds to the endurance of poppers as a powerful symbol. Amyl nitrite shows up in some of the most successful detective fiction on screen and on the page, from Sherlock Holmes to *Murder, She Wrote*. Ampoules of amyl nitrite are even close to Hercule Poirot as he dies alone during an attack of angina.

The novel in which poppers are perhaps most central to a death plot is *Dance: Ten Murder: Maybe?* by Ken Landsdowne. The story in this detective romp makes a little more sense than its title does, and it centres around Jeremy "JB" Bent, a successful mystery novelist. JB is also an avatar for Lansdowne, who appears to have self-published eight books in the Bent Mysteries series from his home in Denver, Colorado. The action in *Dance: Ten Murder: Maybe?* gets going when JB witnesses the death of a Broadway musical director called Teddy Brewster. The deceased appears to have suffered a heart attack, but JB notices "a whiff of something, a smell lingering in the air over Teddy's body". The smell is poppers, and JB knows it. A little later, JB and his pal discuss who would want Teddy Brewster dead, and who would give him poppers. "Kept me awake most of the night," says JB.

The mystery of Brewster's death drives JB all over Manhattan in the mid-1980s, through musical theatres, yellow cabs and parties for lovies. It is a fun world built on top of the author's commentary about air kisses settling disputes and plates studded with canapés, "those odd little combinations of foods on crackers that New York caterers seem to favour. Chutney and rutabaga together anyone?" As a mystery novelist, JB sits alongside Jessica Fletcher from *Murder, She Wrote*, and in an even longer line of amateur sleuths. He is also supremely gay, lusting after the newly deceased producer's "incredibly sexy" son and attending circle jerk parties filled with men in "derrick hats, leather vests, tank tops, and workman boots".

Although JB knows that poppers are used during sex, he also knows what effect they have on the heart. The suspicion running through the plot is that poppers caused Teddy Brewster's death, as a kind of suicide or a murder. Either way, it's serious business, and poppers are linked to the worst of fates. It becomes clear that Teddy liked to live life in the fast lane, with lots of lovers, smoking and partying – and that he was suffering from a brain tumour and a weak heart. Deciding that he would rather die having pleasure by placing stress on his heart, Teddy parties even harder. His doctor tells JB, "He refused all of our advice and went on to actively pursue a completely hedonistic lifestyle."

It turns out that Teddy had asked his sexy son, the one JB fancies and sleeps with, to help him to die. So the son put amyl nitrite in the inhaler his dad used whenever his weak heart struggled. This way, when Teddy felt a heart attack coming on, he could sniff the amyl to make his poor heart work harder than it could manage. That is how he died. JB doesn't even figure this all out, instead he has to wait for the sexy son to confess. In Lansdowne's twisting novel, a man tries to die from pleasure, but it is poppers that finish him off.

There is something similar going on in an episode of *Pose*. This HBO television series is also set in New York City, at roughly the same time as *Dance: Ten Murder: Maybe?* – but in an entirely different world. Far from the white, middle-class musical theatre land of Lansdowne's book, *Pose* is set among the poor, working-class people of colour and transgender people who thrive in their homegrown ballroom nightlife. Many characters are also sex workers, and in the episode entitled "Butterfly/Cocoon" Elektra is working as a dominatrix with a client who likes to wear a gas mask containing poppers. Elektra is out of the room when he dies, so the viewer never really knows how he suffers. Perhaps the liquid went into his mouth and stomach, and then he choked on his vomit inside the gas mask. In *Pose*, the proximity of pleasure and death is tight. It is only relieved somewhat by the dark humour in the rest of the episode, which turns into a caper as Elektra and her girls try to dispose of the body.

In more than one episode of *Murder, She Wrote*, Jessica Fletcher suspects amyl nitrite is the killer's weapon. In an episode of *Columbo* set aboard a cruise ship, the murderer sniffs amyl nitrite in order to induce a mild heart attack in himself. This puts him in the ship's hospital, which is the perfect alibi for him to nip out during the night and shoot a woman before slipping back into his hospital bed. The death plots for poppers are a little more complicated in Holmes and Poirot, but they are still far away from pleasure.

As a Victorian, Arthur Conan Doyle must have heard of amyl nitrite's usefulness in relieving pain caused by heart trouble. In 1893, he wrote about it in the short story "The

Resident Patient", featuring his detective Sherlock Holmes.[8] The story concerns a doctor called Percy Trevelyan who is a known authority on catalepsy, a medical condition where the patient enters a trance or seizure, becoming rigid, and loses their sensation and consciousness. Most of the story is Trevelyan recounting a strange night to Holmes, in which he was visited by two gangsters, one posing as a Russian nobleman suffering from this unnerving condition. The fake patient is elderly, thin and demure, but Trevelyan notes that he was struck more by the companion. As if giving a brief to the poster designer for a gay club night, he tells Holmes, "This was a tall young man, surprisingly handsome, with a dark, fierce face, and the limbs and chest of a Hercules."

Trevelyan is taking notes from the patient when suddenly he notices him sitting bolt upright with a blank face. "I had obtained good results in such cases by the inhalation of nitrite of amyl," he tells Holmes later, "and the present seemed an admirable opportunity of testing its virtues. The bottle was downstairs in my laboratory, so leaving my patient seated in his chair, I ran down to get it." He thinks he was away for no more than five minutes, but when he returns the patient and his hunky companion have vanished. The amyl nitrite is left unused, Trevelyan's experiment left dangling.

The wonder drug lies untouched by Hercule Poirot's bed too, as Agatha Christie's famous detective dies from an angina attack. Earlier in *Curtain*, the last novel published in Christie's lifetime, Poirot is taunted by the murderer he is investigating, who sees him struggling with angina. The man withholds Poirot's amyl nitrite ampoules just as he needs them and even calls our hero an "old man". Poirot eventually retrieves the medicine, and relieves his suffering. The scene serves to show how dastardly this murderer is, but also to show how much Poirot has come to rely on poppers. Later, Poirot kills the murderer to stop him from killing others, and then chooses not to stop his own death when the angina comes on again. Instead, he asks God for forgiveness and succumbs to death. Poirot is found in a foetal position, his hand clutching a rosary.

By not using his amyl nitrite, Poirot suffered and died. In its final moments, the detective's body was far away from pleasure. But the idea of pleasure is kept at a distance from all the bodies in this chapter. Even though the majority of poppers use today, and through much of the twentieth century, was for pleasure, the fictional and even non-fiction representations of the drug have kept that feeling at arm's length.

I would not make a plea for a "fairer" representation of poppers, whatever that might mean. Or even a more "positive" representation. I do not work in PR, marketing or advocacy. If this book is a plea for anything, it is for pleasure – for the time and space to dream about it, to plan for it, to experience it. Those of us who enjoy poppers have to rely on ourselves to focus on pleasure, because the culture that depicts poppers has little space for it. In the Holmes and Poirot stories, amyl nitrite is a medicine, shown to work but also withheld. These are pretty old-fashioned stories by traditional writers who were interested in poisons and medicines as plot devices. Their worlds are dark and oozing with criminality. There is no place for pleasure. And their genres are still popular today, with more recent writers preying on our anxieties. We worry about being murdered or simply being ill. Do we also worry about dying before we have experienced enough of the pleasures our bodies are capable of?

A similar question is raised by those fictions that turn poppers into a weapon, or at least a cause of death, as in Lansdowne's book and *Pose*. These are complicated representations because they portray deaths that are linked with pleasure. Sex and death are an intoxicating mix, as seen in Chapter 4. That's a wonderful dramatic paradox – seek pleasure, find death. There is something biblical about it, as Mother Superior Mary Regina would know. Her use of poppers in *Nunsense* is funny though. Humour joins weaponising as another common use of poppers by writers. In both *Nunsense* and the *Poppers* comic, authors are really poking fun at users. There is no judgement in either case. Even Yves, the comic character who describes poppers use as "disgusting", is portrayed as someone with a rod up his arse. The overall view of poppers in *Poppers* is that they are just a part of life, but really there is something silly about all these pumped-up gay men preening in front of mirrors. They are not shamed for sniffing poppers specifically, but overall, their pursuit of pleasure is seen as a bit daft.

The newspapers and online news websites have a particular market in using poppers to shame people. Gordon Ramsay's story of dipping into a hotel for a sex session with a woman and her three-for-a-tenner poppers is one of many such tales – the rich and famous, doing something sleazy, with the privilege of wealth, luxury and time... These folks do not necessarily need to be celebrated, but why in particular is their pursuit of pleasure something that is decadent or shady? Is it because many of us are jealous of their pleasures? Why can't more of us build sexual pleasure into our days? Why do so many of us push sex until the moment we get into bed, knowing we are tired and unable to enjoy it?

So pleasure plays a lesser role in all the reproductions of poppers above, below humour, shame, medicine and death. Perhaps writers find that pleasure itself is too boring for a story. There are so few stories in mainstream culture that are about the pursuit of pleasure. Usually, pleasure just entices characters into a pursuit of their "real" desire, which is love and romance. The denouement may be happiness, or it may be death, depending on the story. Pleasure is rarely portrayed as a goal in itself, in storytelling. However, in the film *Mes Chéris*, transboi Jamal Phoenix says farewell to his boobs before his mastectomy by enacting a sexual fantasy with them.[9] Phoenix's goal is achieved, and that's the end. The film *Lemon Taste* throws lemons and their bitter juice into moments where characters are cruising, being voyeurs, and hooking up.[10] Both of these queer films manage to centre pleasure and physical sensation. Both are also short, pornographic, and subvert the story expectations that most viewers are used to.

If you want to see poppers used by storytellers in depictions of pure pleasure, you have to watch porn. The little brown bottle often shows up in gay porn especially, and some films depict the performers helping each other to sniff, then their faces flushing as they begin to feel the effect and to slowly move against each other in the bliss of a shared sexual connection. The representation of people sniffing poppers during their filmed sex acts is so different from when they are seen in death dramas or satirical comics. But there is one other place where poppers have been represented as purely pleasurable – parliament.

In 2016, Britain's governing Conservative Party intended to ban poppers, among many other psychoactive substances. The ban would have hampered the victimless pleasures of gay men, and many more. Gays and other humans in the QUILTBAG had long come to expect this kind of thing from Tories. In 1988, they called our relationships "pretended families" in legislation that banned public authorities such as schools from recognising us. But when it came to a bill on banning poppers, in a fabulous use of his privilege as an MP, Crispin Blunt, a Conservative representing Reigate, stood up in the House of Commons to say:

I use poppers. I out myself as a poppers user. And would be directly affected by this legislation. And I was astonished to find that it's proposed they be banned and, frankly, so were very many gay men.[11]

Blunt added that he thought poppers were "perfectly OK", making a plea for pleasure in a surprising venue, and showing something unique to the human spirit. His intervention into a matter of public policy was pretty self-serving, which should not make for the most compelling argument in a parliament. But it did show that one purpose of parliament is to imagine freedom. In Blunt's case, it was the freedom to pursue pleasure. As he made his speech, his Conservative colleague David Davis sat scowling on a green-leather bench to Blunt's rear. To see Davis's facial protest is one of the pleasures of watching a recording of Blunt's speech, maybe because Blunt had no idea about the performance going on behind him.

He may, however, have seen the protest that came after the speech in the form of a homophobic opinion piece from Rod Liddle, a political writer. "I would have thought that the requirement for amyl nitrate [sic] to relax the sphincter muscle and lube to accommodate entry was God's way of telling you that what you're about to do is unnatural and perverse," he wrote after hearing Blunt's speech, adding with all his power of eloquence: "So eeeeuw."[12]

Generating protests from the likes of Liddle and Davis, overnight Blunt became a gay hero, if only for fifteen minutes. In the end poppers were not controlled by legislation any more than they already were. Poppers remain controlled by culture – where they are linked to shame and guilt. Pleasure through poppers, it seems, sits "below" most culture: in porn and in actual use. The feeling is ultimately intrinsic, sensorial, lived. Every time a person lifts a bottle of poppers to a nostril, they seek a pleasure that comes not from any external culture but from inside their own human body.

He's got nipple piercings but he says they don't do much. Maybe cold metal is a poor substitute for touch. I tell him sometimes all I need is to pass my fingertip over my nipple. He has only himself to touch these days, tidied away to avoid the virus in the air outside. We look at each other through our computer screens, and we agree that we're ready.

We configure our viewing experiences. Half the screen is our video call, where I can see his piercings and his shy face, and the other half is our chosen popperbator trainer video. We count down from three, and then hit play in sync. The video starts with a beat and images of men. I see what he's seeing. I see him.

I am watching bodies that are recorded and edited, and I am witnessing a body whose life is unfolding right now. We are sharing a moment. No matter how mundane or fleeting this moment, we are fixing it onto our timelines – and the line stretches ahead of us as we look into each other's bedrooms and wish we were touching each other's skin. The line stretches off the screen, of course, far beyond the timeline on the video that will stop after twenty minutes and fifty-four seconds (when an ad or another video will auto-play).

For now, in our digital, disconnected space, in our solidifying moment, our bodies are potential. I notice him stroke his nipple, and I can hear his reaction in my headphones. And then the video gives us our instruction. GET READY. We lift our little bottles and unscrew. 3... 2... 1... HIT.

Together we inhale.

7. HIT / HOLD / RELEASE

I like design, NPR, hiking, biking, gastronomy, astronomy, synthpop, espresso, and fur – manly fur.

That's the online bio posted by marcotureno, a user of xtube. com, a porn-sharing website. It is a cute list of interests, topped by hairy men. You might not be able to see it, but if you add up the likes in his list you can start to approach his artistic vision. He seems to have made only one video, or at least just one using the name marcotureno. The work is a compilation of porn clips he ripped from existing videos, adding music and words to create something new. The title card contains its date of completion: 20150605. The video is fourteen-and-a-half minutes long and it lives on countless porn websites, ripped, shared, transferred, commented on, viewed and used. Like all porn, the video has a primary purpose of arousing the viewer and helping them to get off. This does not make marcotureno's video distinctive. The thing that makes it distinctive is how the assembled clips and beats are overlaid by words that instruct the viewer to sniff poppers as they watch.

"Time to train your cock," says one of the video's first commands. "All hits are mandatory. Inhale poppers on HIT. Hold in breath on HOLD. Exhale breath on RELEASE."

This is not the kind of thing you hear on marcotureno's beloved NPR, the National Public Radio in the United States. But everything else in his list of likes somehow hints that his work is concerned with the body. Espresso and synthpop stimulate the heart and mind. Hiking and

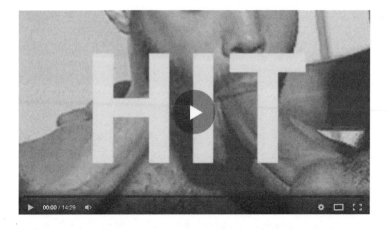

00:00 / 14:29

biking create a life-affirming physical exertion. Design is about manipulating things into something pleasing and useful. Gastronomy is the pleasure of taste. And astronomy – well, let's hold on and together we'll reach the stars.

The list is only a short bio, probably written quickly, to accompany marcotureno's avatar on a porn site. But it is also a recipe for enjoying life from one online video-maker among many who have created the body of work that seeded a sub-culture. These "trainer" videos offer a unique place to use poppers. It is far from the Victorian wards in the Edinburgh Royal Infirmary and the Manhattan dancefloors of the 1970s. The combining of instructions, porn and music into a video that uses the language of training (repetition, submission and endurance) has become a significant part of poppers culture. Porn sites are now filled with videos like marcotureno's (his was not the first). These videos are designed for solo use, often telling the viewer to use headphones to deepen their private immersion into the world of the video. And the viewers even have a name, as marcotureno knew when he wrote the title of his video in 2015: "Trainer compilation for popperbators (only male)".

A bator is a person who wanks a lot, especially one who sees wanking as its own activity. It is not just a way to climax or release. If you think about wanking, if you make plans for it, if you dedicate time to exploring yourself, to trying new pleasures – you are a bator. If you sniff poppers while you wank, as part of your solo sexual practice – you are a popperbator.

Bators also often like to edge themselves close to climax and then stop. Edgers repeat this pattern over and over in order to intensify their eventual orgasm. If you are a bator or an edger who also uses lots of porn, you may be a gooner. Gooners can boast of a porn addiction, especially online. Their avatars compete over how many minutes of porn they have watched and how many orgasms they have had in the past hour. Part of being a gooner is talking about how to structure your life around consuming porn. (There are also online gooner recovery groups.)

So: a bator may edge his way through a session by gooning out on compilation porn and poppers. "Can't wait to get home this eve and find a bro to cam with, huff deep together, encourage each other to go deeper and deeper until we're both a gooning drooling mess," posted one user of popperbate.com, a website for people of the same interests.

The nature of popperbator trainer videos as a collage of clips is especially important. If you don't particularly fancy the body on the screen right now, just wait a moment and a fresh one will take its place. You don't even have to click or skip for that. Clips usually last only a few seconds. Makers also usually assemble these videos into an alluring sequence. In fact, these sequences can be romantic in the way they often track a conventional courtship. A video that particularly targets gay men might go something like this...

Still images, often arty, of men. Looming music, soft beats. A focus on their torsos or arms or bums.

Immediately, these men are sexual objects. Then maybe some slow-moving clips of men touching their bodies, or their dicks still inside their trousers. Maybe some images of faces looking interested in another, or in you. This may soon transition into shots that feature two men, kissing, or touching. The beat picks up, but there are no naked dicks yet. The words have started: instructions to sniff poppers and to touch yourself. And the rhythm drives you on, to the next clip and the next one. As you watch these erotic objects and you feel your first rush, the video-maker has built a world around you. You are in a union with him, and the figures he has assembled just for you.

Clip after clip after clip, transitioning into more and more physical intimacy between the men within them. Soon they are sucking each other. Soon they may be three or more men to a clip. Soon you drift through a sequence of bums and holes and fingers and tongues. You are told to sniff again, and hold, and you hold while the latest clip slows down, and then the maker tells you to RELEASE. As you exhale, he pushes the video on to a new section of harder movements, faster bodies and more rapid editing, snapping from one to the next – and the rush suffuses your body.

The sequences continue, into different penetrations and locations and positions and bodies. And this is how popperbating videos follow a pattern from seduction to climax. Through careful compilation and instructions, the video-maker has controlled your sex life for fourteen-and-a-half minutes. You and he have made a connection of sorts, one solo practice to another, from editing to wanking. And you are continuing something I started when I was about fifteen years old, with two VHS tapes, two VCRs, a SCART cable and some soft-focus erotica I taped off the TV.

I don't have much time. I can never be sure when my family members will arrive home but when they do they might want to know why the VCR is missing from the lounge. It is with me, in my bedroom. I've twinned it to my own private VCR and TV. I'm lucky to have them, and my parents don't even ask any questions about why I do. They just know I like watching films.

I also like wanking a lot, and I like compiling clips of romantic sex scenes. I need the family VCR to do this. I carefully connect everything with a chunky SCART lead. I insert the hefty VHS tapes into their separate machines. I fast-forward through the recorded TV show. When the sex begins, I let it play and hit record on the second VCR. When it stops, usually two minutes later, I hit stop. Then I fast-forward to look for the next scene. This is how I compile a tape of sex.

If I am more enterprising, I could make some money at school. But I am not producing these tapes for others. They are for me, and me alone. They are my secret hobby. They are my shame.

The scenes themselves are soft. They are mostly stolen from erotic TV dramas from the US. One series is called Red Shoe Diaries. *Each episode of this series has the same narrative framework of a different woman answering a personal ad in a newspaper to describe a different story of passion, love, betrayal, that kind of thing. They are played late at night on Channel 5, the only terrestrial station in the UK that is daring enough to broadcast them. I have no interest in the stories. I record them so I don't have to watch them. I just copy the sex scenes over to my compilation. Each episode contains no fewer than two such scenes, no more than three. Every scene features one man and one woman. You always see her breasts and his bum, usually her bum too. You never see their genitals. For me the best shots are the ones where the man is penetrating the woman against a wall or flat on a bed and the angle is such that you can watch his bum flexing. My appetite for these shots is never satisfied.*

But the best clips on my growing compilation tape are those from Queer as Folk, *a comedy drama about three white gay men in Manchester. I dodge the story in these episodes too, as I giddily transfer the kissing shots and the fucking scenes onto my blank VHS. Again, no dicks. Just nipples and bums, but also talk of rimming, and then the actual thing!!!, and then a guy's feet in the air as he lays on his back to get fucked in the bum.*

Soon our family dial-up modem is good enough for more options than the TV can offer. I find images first, loading line by line. Video clips that last twenty seconds – just short enough to be downloaded without overloading the scratchy connection. I assemble these clips into playlists, building digital compilations like my VHS mixtapes. I learn my parents' schedules and I plan my own. I make appointments with myself and the KY Jelly I buy in the shopping centre in Grimsby. I never have much time in the house by myself, but I do make the time – the time to be home, with my tapes, alone.

Some of the scenes I collected and curated as I became a sexual person are still a part of my erotic imagination. I'm a member of the generation that can quote and storyboard *Queer as Folk* scenes from memory. I could describe for you the exact choreographies of some of my blurry digital discoveries, twenty years after I last saw them. I now have to assume that they will stay with me until dementia muddles them.

My endless sequencing of these images, the montages of bodies and sounds, the relentlessness of fucking, the novel couplings, the confusion of locations and angles – all of this is what brought me to popperbator trainer videos.

It would be many years before I would find poppers, or even hear about them. But as a sexual teenager I was definitely a bator. Wanking was a significant part of my life, even though it was entirely secret, never shared, never discussed. I may have talked in vague terms about it with friends, but they didn't know about exactly what I was watching or thinking about. They didn't know about my tapes or my clips. My sex was entirely solo, entirely private. A lot of that privacy is due to my shame of watching men. Perhaps that shame actually dominated my early sexuality. Perhaps that shame held my private world together.

In making my compilations I took control. I overrode the work of performers, producers and editors as I clipped their scenes into my own sequences. With my double-VCR and my private playlists I dominated the viewer – me. I ruled my own wank sessions: my editor-self built a sequence in advance, and then my bator-self followed it. My practice also collected a group of bodies. As figures on a screen, performers who were lit and directed, they were more bodies than people. Sometimes just parts. I omitted their stories. I literally fast-forwarded through everything they went through before sex and after. Years and years after butchering *Queer as Folk*, I finally watched the whole series and realised how many other emotions I had missed out on.

Some people find friends or lovers in this teenage moment, but I trusted only myself. I could not bear to tell a friend or family member about my interests, so I connected with images instead. I found strangers on websites and chat rooms, of course: groups on MSN and Yahoo! where I chatted a little with avatars. Who knows who they were. Their text may have been typed in real time but they were far less real to me than the constructed figures in my clips. I learnt techniques for solo pleasure from a website called jackinworld, and from the age of around fifteen I committed to my practice. If you fast-forward you will find me alone on New Year's Eve in 2017, age thirty-three.

I am sitting on my bed with a bottle of poppers and every intention of finishing by midnight. But I don't get to choose anything for the next little while. The maker of the video that is starting to play is in control. It is the first video of its kind that I have ever seen. Its author is like the teenager I was, editing, sequencing, controlling. Somehow through this video he and I are making contact. He is in charge of what I see, where I touch myself, how long I last – and right now he is telling me to sniff deep.

Among the many innovations of video makers like marcotureno is the one that combines a bator's use of poppers with his need to be told what to do. One thing I realise when I become a popperbator is that poppers and domination go hand in hand. As I arrive into a new realm in my sexuality, it seems that I like to cede control to a person who cut a video with commands for when I should inhale. The same as sniffing poppers, being told what to do can be a relaxing experience. When you sniff, literally parts of your fibre and flesh loosen up. You might even say that the normally taut regulation of your body eases up for a few moments.

Your mind loses some of its control too. That is a common feeling of many drugs, of course. And because the sensation is so short-lived with poppers, it is easy to under-appreciate it. But what happens when you cede some of that control is a submission. And every submission needs a dominator – a dynamic that has a distinctive place in sex between men. (Other bodies play with domination during sex, but here I am only able to talk of the type between bodies that identify as male or as men, or are perceived as such.)

Poppers have been implicated in this ever since Larry Townsend began work on codifying dom/sub practices among gay men in the 1970s. In 1972, he published the first edition of what became a very popular book called *The Leatherman's Handbook*.[1] The book explained everything to do with leather sex and culture. It is not only to do with wearing leather, but also about different roles and specific fetishes. Townsend's book sits on the fulcrum of domination and submission, in which one partner likes to control and the other likes to be controlled. The *Handbook* is not a manifesto for this way of life; more like an encyclopaedia with notes on etiquette. In a section on the leather bar scene and the basic equipment you need if you want to be a part of it, Townsend writes, "A T-shirt or tank top that fits your chest and shows off your firm, slender torso is never out of place. If you don't have a firm, slender torso, or if it's too cold for such light covering, a leather jacket or Levi jacket with a blue workshirt is fine."

He spends many pages going into detail about various leather options, from boots to belts and hats. Whether the leather baby desires to fuck or be fucked, to dominate or submit, he must prepare to "prove his masculinity", says Townsend:

Although this motivation is more readily apparent in a man desiring to be a top, it also holds for a bottom. By placing himself in the position of helplessness and subservience, the M [masochist] is proving he "can take it like a man". The heavier the punishment he can endure, the more this perception is reinforced.

Townsend steers his reader away from scuffed tennis shoes and cologne, and towards cockrings and poppers:

Of course, most guys who use amyl (or butyl) will carry a bottle in their pockets. If you do this, leave it in your pocket while you're in the bar. Most proprietors take a very dim view of people sniffing on their premises, and in some jurisdictions it is illegal to possess.

Poppers, which Townsend calls "amyl" or "sniffs", appear through this handbook. There is a section on what amyl does to the body and why it is used during sex. Updated editions into the 1980s noted the controversy over whether poppers harmed the immune system. Townsend even includes a section in his book on the smells that are and are not part of the leather scene (cologne out, amyl in). "Any of the standard 'sniffs,' especially if they are a bit rancid, smell like old boots. A lot of guys react positively to this," he writes, noting that amyl had been recreational since the 1950s.

In his sexy fiction, Townsend implicates poppers deeper as a drug of domination. He wrote a story called "Kidnapped!", which he published in an edition of *The Leatherman's Workbook* from 1976.[2] That story's narrator is bungled into a van and chained to a chair, blindfolded:

> Before I could answer, or offer any protest, he pulled the zipper shut across my mouth. My fingers closed about the chain, as he placed an inhaler into one of my nostrils, depressing the other to force me to draw breath through the other. I'd sniffed amyl only once before, but the effect had been exciting. Now, it seemed to lift me off the floor... waves of pounding euphoria coursing my veins. "More, punk, more," he whispered. "You're gonna need it! Breathe it in... deep breath, deeper..."

This passage ends with a realisation for the narrator: he is fully submitting to his dom, and doing so with desire. "I really wanted whatever abuse he might decide to inflict upon me." It could be the amyl, or it could be the wine he has been forced to suck off his master's cock. The dom stands at the front of the blinded narrator, forcing him to sniff again as a daddy spoons food into his baby's mouth. And then there is a surprise from behind. "That's right, punk; there's more than just one guy."

Townsend seems to favour the inhaler as a vector for amyl, because it appears in other stories too. In "The Bigot", another short story from 1976, the characters are Gene, who persecutes gays, and Tim, a blond and bearded leatherman. Kidnapping is also a common motif in Townsend, so Tim captures Gene and, in an act of vengeful power reversal, makes him inhale amyl from a "silver bullet". Gene rides the high and the sensations in the room. "With the hood no longer in place to mute his sense of hearing, the throbbing rise and fall of music surrounded him – Mahler, Tim had told him later."

Townsend's sexy shorts are just porn before we had popperbator trainer videos. I'm yet to find a popperbator video with Mahler on the soundtrack, though. Usually it's techno or dark synthpop. For me, the music is hugely influential in my enjoyment of these videos. I have discovered some favourite bands, like TR/ST, when their pirated tracks have turned up in my life in this way. Just as this music spills out from a porn session into my life in general, domination and submission are not just to do with sex. The dynamic is a way of life for many people.

In *Box Hill*, a novel by Adam Mars-Jones from 2020 but set in 1975, Colin is a submissive who literally trips over Ray as he naps under a tree, tumbling out of his parents' home and into Ray's. He submits to Ray's authority because he needs to. He needs authority, or a carer at least, someone to make him feel that he is worth something. Ray, of course, is looking for the flip-side. This is what ties them together. Their entire relationship is structured around the power dynamic. As soon as Colin moves in, Ray throws Colin's toiletries in the bin. "He didn't want me to smell of anything but myself, that was pretty clear," Colin tells the reader. If only Colin had read *The Leatherman's Handbook*, he might have spared Ray the trouble.

Ray also asserts his authority by withholding a key from Colin, so he can control his movements, and by making him sit naked on the floor when Ray's friends come round to play cards. There is a tense scene where it is established that Ray is happy to share his boy with the rest of the gang, and another where Ray demonstrates to them that it is he who ultimately owns Colin. The relationship is consensual and not abusive… Mars-Jones's project is to explore why a person can live as a submissive. It is almost satirical, but really it is tragic. The novel is subtitled "A Story of Low Self-Esteem".

There is a similar dynamic in "The Little Saint" by Garth Greenwell, a story in his book *Cleanness*. The nameless narrator cruises online and finds someone who describes himself as a "no limits whore" available to anyone who wants to fuck him rough. The story describes their hook-up in the kind of sublime pornographic detail that characterises Greenwell's work. The narrator has cast himself as the dominant, but he is sometimes so surprised at the submissive's willingness that he has to be nudged back into character.

He does get it though. Just about. When the sub begins to stroke himself, the dom tells him to stop. "I had spoken sternly," he says, "but I was glad to see it, that he was so eager, that he was enjoying himself." Greenwell's dom doesn't realise this here, but thinking about the sub's pleasure means that he has not really taken the full control required by his role. Later, when the sub is sucking the dom's dick, the dom tells his reader, "he was the best I ever had, and I gave myself over to it, over to him, I forgot the role I was supposed to play and let him do whatever he wanted". Later still, the dom becomes more and more active, more controlling, which involves taking the sub's head in his hands and fucking his face. He uses him like an object.

The sub sometimes uses language from porn videos, and the dom joins in eventually. Greenwell's narrator thinks of these exchanges as "inane dialogue", an admission that they connect through pre-ordained roles. And as they fuck harder and harder, the dom says words that he had heard as a little boy. Faggot, he calls the sub, you dirty faggot. The sub admits he is nothing, and the dom says he is nothing. The scene crescendos here, as a porn video would, into a joint orgasm. They have matched through domination and submission, forces that can only connect because they require each other. When the dom finally settles into his role, becoming fully active and denigrating the sub, the connection is made, the climax reached.

But, unlike in porn, there is a coda, when the dom starts to weep. Greenwell's perfect prose leads the reader to understand at the same moment as the dom that he feels just like the sub. In becoming the dom he had pulled on the cloak of the awful man, probably his dad, who had always made him feel ashamed. It takes the re-enactment of this trauma for the characters somehow to transcend it, although the story is not conclusive about that. Greenwell is far more interested in the ambiguity of a scene like this than in claiming something about dom/sub psychology.

Whatever a reader's interpretation of his characters' desires to play roles, what Greenwell does is portray a union of two people. When I read "The Little Saint" and other stories by Greenwell, I think about the way his characters pursue their desires with others, even discreetly. I think about this because, for me, for so many years, I pursued mine alone. This meant wanking privately – in the way it is usually viewed, as a solo indulgence. In fact, we often see wanking as anti-social. It is even more solitary than reading because at least with reading you can acceptably discuss your favourite book with a colleague. You can even share and swap. Wanking is far more private. It is why we feel we're transgressing when we do talk about it. It is why I felt shame for so many years about it. Even the most sexually free person knows the difference between talking openly about how they make their coffee and how they wank.

Of course, this privacy is a cover for what's actually going on. Wanking is not really a private act at all. People do it with friends or siblings as they're growing up, showing, learning, testing, sharing. Partners do it together, sometimes over long distances. Men in particular meet in parks and toilets to watch each other do it, especially if they are too afraid to touch each other. And online, strangers meet in live video rooms, dozens of people wanking together in the twenty-first century's answer to the dark rooms and sex clubs of the 1970s. Some of them keep their faces out of the frame. The effect is a wall of fleshy boxes, each featuring a different body, a different technique, different tastes. They may have different tastes but, in fact, they have the same desire in that moment – to be together. An online live video room filled with dozens of wanking bodies is the apex of bator culture. It is a solo practice made communal. It is a profoundly social experience because the bators' bodies are experiencing the same sensations at the same time – just as spectators at a football game or family members dancing at a wedding party.

So bating online is social, and it is also humane. A video room or a chat forum largely omits things like the amount of money a bator has, or their religion, their sexuality, their gender, their job... Only their body is visible. Sometimes conversation is taken up by talk of endurance tinged with masculinity, but thankfully conversation is minimal anyway. I'm sure that many bators in these spaces are sometimes made to feel uncomfortable because of their skin tone, weight or disability. But these rooms seem to include far more body types, with far less labelling, than professional porn videos do.

Bators in these spaces are doing the same thing observed by Samuel Delany, a writer and pervert, when he cruised New York City's cinemas and dark rooms. "Given the mode of capitalism under which we live," he wrote in 1999, "life is at its most rewarding, productive, and pleasant when the greatest number of people understand, appreciate, and seek out interclass contact and communication conducted in a mode of good will."[3]

Delany knew that interclass contact has to be one of society's most important aims. Only if we experience the humanity of another, even someone whose life is so different to our own, can we build a fair society. So when it is in the back row of the cinema or a Zoom room, wanking is communal, not self-indulgent or anti-social. Bators settle down into their desk chairs, open a video call, begin to touch themselves and see others do the same – and through this communion, which extends from their own fibres through their broadband cables, they create a shared utopia.

I do not mean to say that I think the world would be wonderful if everyone sat alone wanking over the internet with others. Different strokes for different folks. The point here is that even the act that we regard as the most private, the most personal, the most anti-social, is actually performed together. Every one of those bators in a box on a shared video call is getting off privately, but really they are doing so in connection to others. Every one of them is here because they want to connect.

I am here because I want to connect. Sometimes when I watch porn I click on a new video, and then on another, and so on, and I wonder if I simply need to interact with something, with someone, to get a feeling. Is my act of clicking, clicking, clicking just a moment of interaction in an otherwise passive state? In a Zoom room there is no clicking because interaction is happening, and now. But I prefer trainer videos for popperbators like me, where I also don't need to click around. In these, another person is already with me – he has curated this stream of images and sounds, and he is speaking to me, and here I am on my bed in the dark responding, sniffing, touching, cumming when he says so.

I marvel at his work. I find his profile, I read about his interests, I find others who make similar videos, I follow them, subscribe to them, submit to them when their new videos arrive. I follow them when they are kicked off pornhub.com. Wherever they find space, these video-makers are building a world, and there are popperbators like me who I enter it with. We share what we like. We meet on cams. Someone even begins a database of popperbator trainer videos in a public Google Sheet, with categories and descriptions to help a bator who is looking. Other bators contribute to the database, of course, commenting on the work of those who make the trainer videos. There is a real fandom for their work. We discuss it, and that brings us together across oceans. We are the dom and the sub in Greenwell's story. We can transcend our shame, because we are the same.

I may have dominated myself with my own compilations when I was fifteen. I may have kept myself secret for years and years. But now I can say I am a bator, and so is he, and he, and he. I can rely on others now – artisan porn compilers with sharp skills in video editing and the need to reach an audience of people like them. I can be fifteen again, but not alone this time.

It is understood among bators that each trainer video requires days and days of work. They have to rip the clips that will make the compilation, build the sequence, write the script, add the graphics, and find the right music.

They blend these elements together to match the bator's experience of feeling the poppers rush. Some makers might give up after one, as marcotureno did. It is impossible to earn money from these videos really, not least because they largely comprise material whose copyright is owned by others. Other makers go on and on, producing more and more, building their audiences. They are not doing this for money.

These artists are building their own sexual utopias, filling them with the bodies, actions and music they like. They know that a viewer who sniffs poppers is more likely to join the fantasy with them, to feel like they are inside it, even just for a few seconds. But then they will issue a new instruction to sniff anyway, and fresh images, and a driving beat. This is how the dom and the sub, the artist and the viewer, can sustain their connections.

In controlling their viewer, popperbator trainer videos sit within the dom/sub culture that Townsend explained in his handbook in 1972. These videos may look self-indulgent and mad. Dom/sub dynamics may seem inhumane. But we are all just trying to reach one another. Domination is one method but it is not required. Plenty of bators meet just to huff and wank together, as they might also meet for a pint in the pub. We are a social species, and we seek to connect with each other. This is why marcotureno completed his profile on xtube.com with his interests in hiking and espresso. He wanted to share something with others, not just his perfect trainer video. He reached millions of individuals in their own little boxes, watching, sharing, discussing, cumming together.

I stopped dancing just before I became a teenager. I withdrew from Stage One, a club for kids who performed musicals in Grimsby. I went to school in my uniform, put my head down, and tried to pass.

I must have believed that it was bad to be one of the gay boys, or associated with them. I must have worried that to be a man I'd have to like fighting and football.

These ideas are like cyanide, which binds to human cells and blocks their oxygen. Without oxygen our cells cannot survive. At the atomic level, cyanide stops us from being.

Who put this poison inside me?

8. Antidote

It's funny that some people are wary of inhaling poppers, because we're already full of poisons. I'm not talking about the microplastics we ingest when we eat fish. I mean the ideas we absorb that make us hate ourselves.

We first have to deal with these poisons when we're teenagers. For most of us this is the first time in our lives when we realise how much free will we have, even if others would force us to feel otherwise. The condition of being a teenager is one of finally being able to make choices about how to live in a shitty world. Jenny Valentish chose to stride through Slough with a bottle of poppers "clanking away in my army satchel alongside the quarter-bottle of vodka". It was the 1990s, and Jenny was a hardcore teenager. At school, she coached people to dip their cigarettes in a bottle of amyl (which is flammable). And on a visit to her elder brother who had made it to university, she introduced him and his housemates to poppers. "The admiration in their eyes as they staggered about the dance floor at the student union indie disco was beautiful to behold," she wrote in her book about addiction, *Woman of Substances*. "I was a legend among men."

Valentish had suffered sexual abuse when she was just seven, "the moment that shame hotwire[d] my brain". Due to her teenage partying with sex and drugs she was negatively branded a slut. By seventeen the only thing she could do was to turn this label into a persona. She began to write and publish *Slapper,* her own music magazine that chronicled her hard-drinking and promiscuous encounters with bands and their publicists. Having accepted the only category placed on her, she realised later that she was a "baby misogynist who was defiantly, desperately one of the blokes".

The thing about realising you have agency is that you also realise that others have it too, and they will use it to stamp on your neck unless you move first. Valentish absorbed the poison of misogyny, the societal and often personal hatred of women. When she sniffed poppers, crashed press junkets and snarled about it all in *Slapper*, she was both absorbing the poison of misogyny while also seeking an antidote to it.

Valentish is the kind of anarchist I stayed the fuck away from when I was a teenager. I didn't like rule-breakers, I didn't like bravado, and I definitely didn't like drugs. I read books and talked to friends and watched sci-fi and waited an hour for my twenty-second porn clips to download. I was becoming a gay man, of sorts, and yet I didn't identify with what I thought the words "gay" and "man" meant. Especially in combination. Rather than acting out like Valentish did, I just lived with my poisons. When the other kids called me a puff or a boff – the supposed shame of being either gay or studious – I mostly just got on with my work.

I tried to pass. I felt ashamed. I thought that gays cared only about nightclubs, sex and their own reflection. I must have picked up this image from somewhere. I was terrified of HIV too, and I associated it with gay sex and death. It was the late 1990s and early 2000s, and I was poorly informed. I should have just been sniffing poppers, but instead I was in crisis. I did not want to be a man if it meant *that,* or a gay if it meant *this*.

When you think of people like Valentish and me, you might think we should be looking for somewhere or some way to be free. She did move countries later, escaping domestic violence, and I landed in London. These relocations may have helped us as individuals to live with our poisons. But people had been trying to eradicate them on our behalf long before they bonded to our cells.

For example, thanks to the activists who splashed fake blood in the offices of pharma companies, HIV drugs became more available and HIV became a more manageable condition. Lesbians had leapt into a BBC studio during a live news broadcast and shouted "Stop Section 28!". They were protesting the legislation that stopped teachers and librarians from mentioning anything to do with being gay. (The law was enacted in 1988, just as I started school, and repealed in 2003, only after I'd left.) A sixteen-year-old called Richard Desmond had anonymously sued the British government to claim his right to have gay sex. He lost, but others tried again and won. Jackie Forster had co-founded a social group and publication for lesbians, then made television news reports and even programmes about being a lesbian despite deep hostility. Streetwise queers in New York City had risen up against police violence at the Stonewall Inn. Peter Wildeblood had stood up against Britain's homophobic establishment, gone to prison and later helped to change the law. Every one of these pioneers had relied on the courage of Karl Heinrich Ulrichs, who was perhaps the first person to describe his gayness as just a part of who he was. Since Ulrichs' speech in 1867, being gay could be seen as an identity, and it became a powerful way of gaining respect and rights. *I am who I am.*

However, for me as a teenager, being a gay man was a negative identity. This darkness is still hard to understand, but now I get a thrill every time I flip a light on it and say how great it is to be gay. This is how "pride" became the slogan for people of sexual and gender difference. Our classic journey is to accept our difference as part of our identity, and assert our pride out on a march or at home in the mirror. Everyone who is queer, undecided, intersex, lesbian, transgender, bisexual, asexual and/or gay – that is, everyone in the QUILTBAG, which is the best way to bunch us if you have to – goes through their own journey. It's an interior journey, with each of us hoping to inhabit queer utopia. And it's an exterior, political journey too, asserted through marches and legislative change. Oppression, shame, self-definition, acceptance, pride. This liberation is the basis of all the dreams of the people of sexual and gender difference.

The 1970s were a particularly dreamy time for those who lived in the QUILTBAG. In this period many of them got together to sniff poppers and describe utopias where everyone was free. I want to share just three of these visions. It still feels necessary to hold each of them in mind today as ideas for a better life. First is the Gay Liberation Front manifesto from 1971, in which that radical group saw itself

> as part of the wider movement aiming to abolish all forms of social oppression.... Women's liberation, black peoples and other national minorities, the working class, young people who are rejecting the bourgeois family and the roles and lifestyles offered them by this society, peoples oppressed by imperialism.[1]

Second is an excerpt from the verdant dreamscape envisaged by Larry Mitchell in his book *The Faggots and their Friends Between Revolutions*. Mitchell set up a company to publish the book in 1977 because no publisher wanted it. The book mixes poetry and prose, manifesto and observation, words and illustration (by Ned Asta). In one episode we find the radical queer men, known as fairies, at home on the land:

> The great gardens of the fairies prosper. The fairies worship their plants and they grow and bear abundant food. In the afternoon, they sing and chant and weed. As the sun cools

they make love with each other, surrounded by tomatoes and marigolds. At night they sleep curled around the cucumbers or intertwined in the beans or covered by the corn. When they awake in the cool mornings, they stroke the plants and give them food. And sometimes the fairies are so overcome with love and passion that they lie in the watermelon patch and masturbate.[2]

Third is the revolutionary statement issued by the Black feminist women who comprised the Combahee River Collective in 1977:

We believe that the most profound and potentially most radical politics come directly out of our own identity, as opposed to working to end somebody else's oppression. In the case of Black women this is a particularly repugnant, dangerous, threatening, and therefore revolutionary concept because it is obvious from looking at all the political movements that have preceded us that anyone is more worthy of liberation than ourselves. We reject pedestals, queenhood, and walking ten paces behind. To be recognized as human, levelly human, is enough.

[...] If Black women were free, it would mean that everyone else would have to be free since our freedom would necessitate the destruction of all the systems of oppression.[3]

The individuals in the collective knew that simply because of who they were they faced oppression in their native USA. They also knew that the strands of who they were (Black, woman and, for some, lesbian) were woven together because a single human being is made of many things. And finally, they knew that these interlocking categories were also the shackles placed on them by the white, patriarchal supremacy that ruled their country. So the bold claim in their statement was that there is no liberty for all until these most maligned identities are free.

Today when I read these three powerful visions the cyanide leaves my cells. I get the rush of oxygen that feels like freedom. But I know that these three ideas are still dreams, decades after they were first presented to the world. Many people remain unconvinced even by the argument from 1867 in which Ulrichs basically said of gay people, "We're fine, please leave us alone". In more than seventy countries in the world, laws criminalise aspects of being a person of gender or sexual difference. All countries and many cultures are home to people who are hostile to gender and sexual freedom. Countless brave activists are fighting these ideas and laws, and they still draw on Ulrichs' thought, as well as the three visions above.

The thinkers behind those three passages were showing us a better time and place for us all to live, where our minds and bodies are freer. I like to think of Larry Mitchell writing that passage about the fairies and the cucumbers, thinking of teenagers like me in the future, hoping that his words and Asta's pictures would reach us and make us realise our options, our potential. It's sad that I didn't find their book until much later, when a friend gave it to me for my thirty-sixth birthday. Mitchell's fairies were based on the very real radical faeries who live in queer communes in the countryside. In that sense, his ideas were very concrete, not just a dream; they were already happening. The ideas of the Combahee River Collective and the Gay Liberation Front were different for being more overtly hopeful. All three visions, whether realistic or not, are grounded in categories that seek to externalise the complex identities of their subjects. Their authors know that a social and political utopia is a dream, but it seems possible when you base it on the strands of feeling and being that weave together in unique ways to make each of us who we are – our identities.

In writing down their visions, they tried to encapsulate identities into words and categories, such as "working class", "fairies", and "Black women". Although these are all incredibly important and powerful categories that mean a lot to the people who use them to describe themselves, no word can come close to expressing the complexity of who a person is, or the *truth* of their *identity*. Words are never enough.

When I think about my teenage angst, the fear of the sexual and gender categories is greater than of my identity. That is because, I believe, identity is a feeling. Identity is an interior experience that, through the spread of certain words and ideas, has also become shared public knowledge. Identity is the person I feel I *am*. Identity is inside me; words and categories like "gay" and "man" are just projections that help me to explain myself to the world. As the poisons of homophobia and patriarchy were doing their best to attack me, I wish I had known about those three visions for better societies. They might have pointed me to a utopia: a place to imagine where I would be free, where the categories wouldn't matter because the Combahee women would have ensured that we'd spotted "all the systems of oppression", and shattered them. But I turned sixteen in 2000, and we hadn't yet reached the Combahee women's utopia. The categories of "gay" and "man" still had meaning, and I felt them in my bones with fear and panic. I hated it when people said I wasn't the right kind of man, and I hated the idea that there was such a thing even more. I kept my desires so secret even when I was dying to talk about them. I realise now that I was looking to be free of these poisons, and that is how I edged towards sci-fi.

The visions of writers who bend space and time have been just as powerful to me as the statements of political actors like those quoted above. And although I'd watched Tony Blair march into Downing Street through crowds of

Union Jack wavers when I was twelve, my introduction to politics really came a year later when I began to watch *Star Trek*. The thing about *Star Trek*, like all art, is the subjective experience that it gives the viewer. As with identity, feeling is a better way of approaching utopia than thinking is. Would I have found utopia in the rational words of the Gay Liberation Front if I had read them as a teenager? Or New Labour's manifesto? Probably not. Instead, I found a utopia through feeling the same experiences as the characters in sci-fi. When Jean-Luc Picard fought the Borg as they tried to assimilate people into their clan of cyborg automatons, I felt the power of recognising my individuality. When Morpheus confirmed Neo's suspicions that real life was really just a simulation called the Matrix, I felt the power of free thinking. I can't even begin to express my feelings about Laura Dern in *Jurassic Park*.

I realise it now – these fictions gave me a way of thinking. Specifically, they even helped me to think about myself, and the future I might want to build. My love of these sci-fi stories is not because "I saw myself represented in them". It is based on their ability to surface the feelings and ideas that I was experiencing inside me. I was particularly attracted to the United Federation of Planets in *Star Trek* as a political union based on equality, diversity and inclusion. (This stated fictional ideal has never been fully realised by the very real humans who've made the shows, hamstrung as they are by the social trappings of the twentieth and early twenty-first centuries.) In *Star Trek*, I saw people of difference living together: humans and Ferengei and Vulcans. I saw freedom from money. I saw ultimate respect for science and exploration. I saw gender parity: women who were as smart and various as the ones I knew in real life, and men who had outgrown earthly ideas of masculinity. I also saw cool spaceships with zappy bits and machines that can manifest whatever drink you ask for.

The humans of *Star Trek* are represented as free and, it seems, living in a utopia. The creator of this universe was a man named Gene Roddenberry, a former US fighter pilot who flew missions in the Second World War. As with the USA, the forces that Roddenberry put into keeping the United Federation of Planets going as an ideal are actually not so desirable. All the *Star Trek* series and films have shown that the Federation maintains peace through war and political interference, often in the name of science and development. Underpinning the Federation, and *Star Trek* as an entertaining exposition of politics, is the idea that we can engineer an ideal world. In fact, the idea that any one group of people comes up with to create an ideal world is a profoundly arrogant one. One person's idea of an ideal world bulldozes through another's. The British Empire tried to establish an ideal world through "civilisation", the revolutionaries in France and Russia through equality and solidarity, the Nazis through racial purity. When you try to build your ideal world, you always spill blood.

Star Trek often dramatises this pattern well, but a certain idea of freedom (Western, liberal) always wins. Even though I enjoy watching *Star Trek*, it doesn't feel like it offers a utopia, really, or a way to live free of our poisons. At least it poses questions, like all good art. But thank the gods for books. Less inhibited than TV, sci-fi books like Ursula Le Guin's *The Left Hand of Darkness* have exploded how I thought about being a man or a male. In that book the alien characters have no gender until they are aroused, when they take one form or another, and each time this happens it could be a different set of sex/gender characteristics.

For those of us who never felt like we were getting our sexuality or gender quite right, that is an extremely exciting idea. And it led me to a spaceship of ultimate freedom: the one captained by Iain M. Banks in his series of sci-fi novels depicting a civilisation known as the Culture. Banks' project with the Culture books was to imagine a post-scarcity society even more futuristic than Roddenberry's. He started with artificial intelligence machines that run everything. These machines are benign, which is an innovation itself in sci-fi where the convention is that robots and software become tyrants. In the Culture, everybody gets everything they need because nothing costs anything to produce and distribute. There is no real crime or harm. Laws are unnecessary, so there are none. Banks described the Culture as a state of utopian anarchy.

Bodies are free, knowing neither shame nor fear. The people of the Culture take a very 1970s approach to fucking: it is various and frequent. They change sex, often back and forth, express their gender as they wish, and even have glands that secrete whatever substance they need to enhance their day. Imagine having that body modification. Imagine not having to wrestle with the safety cap on the poppers bottle during sex to make sure you keep the bottle upright so you don't spill flammable liquid over your lover's nipples. Instead, you can just secrete the fumes from your glands directly into your bloodstream.

This is just one freedom you'd have if you lived in the Culture. The possibilities are endless. In the novel *Matter* from 2008, the character Djan Seriy Anaplian grows up in a feudal society before leaping into space to join the Culture:

[S]he started to notice that although there was near infinite physical variety here, there was no deformity, and while there was prodigious eccentricity, no dementia. There were more facial, bodily and personality types than she could have imagined, but they were all the product of health and choice, not disease and fate. Everyone was, or could be if they so desired, beautiful in both form and character.

Anaplian accepts some pretty decent enhancements to her own body. Among them are fingernails that can lase to signal, blind or kill, and a tiny reactor in her skull that can keep her conscious for years if she is starved of oxygen. As she transitions from class-based medievalism to the ultimate tech paradise in space, she finds she has more choices. In fact, infinite choices. What the Culture offers above all else is the freedom to choose. This feels enormously powerful, of course, especially in relation to Anaplian's backward family. "She felt, she realised one day, like a god."

Having a godlike amount of choice brings a problem. When you can choose to do anything, to *be* anything, who are you? The people of the Culture have absolute choice in everything, so it is hard to know who they really are. Without constraint, what creates and defines your identity? When we think about our own lives, our sense of self comes from the choices we make within the constraints we are born into. If we live without constraints, how do we even *learn* who we are?

I'm not saying that constraints are good for us and we should keep them. Of course, it is right that here on Earth in the twenty-first century we emancipate each other along the lines proposed by the Combahee River Collective and the Gay Liberation Front. They offer a blueprint for a utopia, a vision and a promise. And they have set us on the path towards it by passing one milestone after another: legal equality, visibility, social acceptance, Lady Gaga, and so on. This kind of utopia will be founded on rights and, because we live under consumerism, goods and services. But all these things are only possible because of the concrete categories we are said to inhabit. These categories are founded in our feelings of identity.

An identity is who you feel you are. That feeling is inexpressible, at least until we live in a telepathic utopia like the one in *Mind of My Mind*, a sci-fi novel by Octavia Butler. No one is inside your head, so how can they know who you really are? How can they know exactly how all your characteristics, experiences, tastes and desires are blended together to make up the feeling of being you? They cannot. All you can do is to help them, by using words with shared definitions such as "gay", "man", "British", "Trekker" – even "queer" although that label at least has ambitions to be an anti-label. Categories are mere fictions, but they are crucial; they are the only way that the visionary writers quoted above were able to be understood.

When millions of people stood up in the middle of the twentieth century and said the category "gay" or "lesbian" about themselves, they could finally see each other. They were no longer alone, like Ulrichs had been on his podium in 1867. They amassed in cities like London and New York. They became groups that businesses could market to. The gay men, in particular, became a demographic whose desires could be targeted with pec-tastic poppers advertisements drawn by artists like Skipper who huffed as he drew. (In their beautiful human complexity, bisexual and pansexual people were harder to target...)

Categories help activists and legislators too. When enough people believe in the shared definitions of sexual categories, they can be protected in law. You need words in order to write a law, and I'm grateful to words for their role in that. But they are only words. I'm happy to describe myself as a gay man, if that description protects me from hate crimes, and helps me to find pubs and lovers. At the same time, I have to accept that there is a limit to the utility of these categories. They are fictions, really. They discourage imagination. They describe me, but don't *define* me – that is what people say when they're trying to explain the difference between a category and an identity. We often constrain ourselves within a certain category for years more than we should, just because we want to be consistent. Freedom from this would help not just people of sexual and gender difference, but also the most heterosexual, gender-conforming person too.

When people name their sexual identity, I think they are really talking about their sexual category. The category, or sexuality, is a useful tool, but it narrows the aperture of what we are able to dream. The endless categorisation and sub-categorisation of porn videos on websites like xtube.com and PornHub enables us to find the fucks we want to watch. Once I found the category of "popperbator" videos, as described in Chapter 7, I lost a weekend. But of course, those images and sounds are just projections, literally leaping off a digital device and into my brain. Do they match exactly what my brain would generate if I left it to its *own* devices? This is one limit of many in pornography; it is a call to consume more expansively. When we press beyond the limits of a category, we find we have very promiscuous desires and erotic imaginations. What you might find sexy may sit just outside your field of vision, and it may surprise you. That is your sexual identity; inexpressible, known only to you, and definitely not a dropdown on PornHub.

Thanks to legislators' use of human categories that describe things like gender and sexuality, or protected characteristics, people like me are freer than Ulrichs was. Although progress is not linear and prejudiced speakers are always seeking to hold us back, we are edging closer towards the utopian anarchy of the Culture. I can only dream of the various things that women, people of colour and QUILTBAGgers would do given the freedoms and modifications afforded them in the Culture (fingernails that can lase to kill?!). In fact, it is the project of the Culture books to explore how people behave when they have freedom. If this is the first time you've heard about the Culture books you might assume them to be boring, filled with characters lazing on space clouds and drinking MDMA-laced piña coladas. But Banks' books are stories, so they need conflict. Conflict happens at the edges of the Culture, when utopian anarchy clashes with other forms of civilization like the medieval ones on Anaplian's homeworld – all because the people in the Culture have an identity crisis. With so much freedom, they don't know who they are. So all they can do is to promote their way of living, using agents to interfere with "lesser" civilisations, sparking wars. It's all very thrilling. It's hard to read about people with lots of freedom interfering with others and not think of rich white gays telling their fellow gays in poor, post-colonial countries how to be free. The only choice left for some "utopias", it seems, is to conquer others.

If one effect of having freedom is to promote our ways of living, another is grounded more in our identities. It seems that the more freedom we have, the more we are interested in who we are. In the past, my gay ancestors found each other in certain places for people who shared the same sexual category. Today we assemble ourselves into ever smaller and tightly defined online groups. We seek out the content made specifically for us, thanks to the artificial intelligence algorithms at Netflix and Instagram. Sometimes we become a little obsessed with the past, preserving the good things that have built our categories today. This is one reason why many people in the QUILTBAG, including me, are fascinated by queer history.

I sometimes wonder how individuals in the QUILTBAG would fare if one day the category-based structure of our modern lives dissolved. Imagine if we all just suddenly deleted the word "heterosexual", forgot what men and women are supposed to be like, and lost our passports. We would start over, trying to find each other, searching for solidarity – but I bet the words coined and alliances forged would differ from the ones we have today. How can that be possible? Because categories can only ever be an approximation of an individual's identity. Because the categories we connect with are contingent on time, place, society, customs. We know this because queer performers from the future have told us.

I'm thinking about Luis Amália and Jade Pollard-Crowe from previous chapters, but also about the musician and producer SOPHIE. SOPHIE held back most forms of identity for years, never showing face, using others' voices, unsettling the ways we rely on physicality to experience one another. SOPHIE even shunned all personal pronouns, and in this way and many others seemed to transcend us all. Music became SOPHIE's chosen method of communication and self-expression.[4] And it was bloody good. Every track is a pristine teardrop filled with human emotions. They sound like something one of the Culture's quantum computers might produce given unlimited processing power.

In the euphoric rhythms of the song "Immaterial", SOPHIE removed the things that we use to categorise ourselves:

Without my legs or my hair
Without my genes or my blood
With no name and with no type of story
Where do I live?
Tell me, where do I exist?

I think SOPHIE existed simultaneously in our minds and our futures. Through producing music that was so full of pleasure, SOPHIE brought an identity to the surface, and was thus able to live fluidly and freely in the Culture, writing lyrics that told us so:

I could be anything I want
Immaterial boys, immaterial girls
Anyhow, anywhere, any place, anyone that I want

But in January 2021 SOPHIE died falling from a balcony when trying to photograph the Moon. SOPHIE was a visitor from the future who will forever be reaching into space. Inside SOPHIE's words, performances and final act is the queer utopia of always grasping, always dreaming of a freer life. The music SOPHIE left behind is an expression of one person's pure identity, as opposed to categorisation, immune to poisons. You might call it soul.

Let SOPHIE be our guide to queer utopia. I don't mean a destination or even a time. I mean a feeling. Queer utopia is the feeling that your body is yours, it's free and full of potential, and it's not poisoned by anyone or their ideas.

Our categories, our shame, our stigmas – they are all poisons, and they act like cyanide. When cyanide enters a human body, its atoms react with the cells in a way that stops them from using oxygen. When cells can't get oxygen, they die, so that is why cyanide is so dangerous to people. Poisoning a person with cyanide first causes a headache and dizziness, then a fast heart rate, and shortness of breath. Within minutes, you get seizures, your heart rate drops, you lose consciousness, and then you have a cardiac arrest. These are the horrors that our poisons do to us, as individuals and as societies. So finding a way to approach queer utopia is the same business as finding an antidote to our poisons.

Poppers cannot remove these poisons, but amyl nitrite actually does counteract cyanide. It is one of several substances that can cause the cyanide atoms to react differently with the atoms in a person's body in a way that is far less harmful to them. It's really magic. Here is a report from 1956 in a journal for pharmacists:

A thirty-nine-year-old man who was in charge of a manufacturing process involving a chemical reaction in a tank inhaled hydrogen cyanide gas from a leaking gasket.

His foreman, being familiar with the management of cyanide poisoning, carried the victim to the open air, administered amyl nitrite by inhalation, and sent for the works doctor.[5]

After a few minutes and a few additional treatments, the man came round. His foreman had kept amyl nitrite in a poisons kit so that one day it could save a life. Before the development of other antidotes, including those specifically formulated to handle cyanide poisoning, kits containing amyl nitrite seem to have been common.

So common, in fact, that their contents have been vulnerable to theft. In 1983, a doctor from the Baton Rouge Chemical Dependency Unit wrote to the *Journal of the American Medical Association* to tell his peers to check emergency treatment kits like the one used by the foreman above.[6] The doctor, Louis Cataldie, had learnt that ampoules of amyl nitrite were regularly stolen from such kits, presumably by people who knew of how good it felt to sniff when you weren't being poisoned. The substance has even been nicked more recently. In 2015, a nurse in Northern Ireland pleaded guilty to stealing seven boxes of amyl nitrite from his workplace.[7]

Even though the substance was present in that nurse's hospital, it is no longer the first choice for the treatment of anything. Although people find their ways, and perhaps that is what the nurse was up to. One person told me that sniffing poppers while he self-administers EMDR therapy, or eye movement desensitisation and reprocessing, has helped to ease him out of enduring traumas. The nitrites are a versatile therapy. The one problem they have historically eased is the one that seems far away from today's associations of the substance: period pain. In the first edition of Martindale's *Extra Pharmacopoeia* in 1883, and many subsequent, period pain (dysmenorrhoea) is listed among the various ailments that amyl nitrite is good for.[8] In 1906, the obstetric physician Amand Routh told an audience at the Charing Cross Hospital in London that he used amyl nitrite as a relief from period pain, especially when "the patient feels chilly".[9]

This treatment seems to have fallen out of use. Pleasure and sphincter relaxation have become the dominant reasons for industrial manufacture of nitrites. But that transition was not inevitable; it is just that the businessmen who built companies around what became known as poppers decided to recognise only distinct uses and categories of user. They may have missed the opportunity to develop a product for people struggling with period pain. Perhaps the poppers industry became so focused on one demographic category that it missed another. Maybe transgender men who have periods could lead an expansion of the poppers market.

Among brands like Throb Hard, XL Gold and Horse Power, there remains a distinctly manly whiff to the marketing of poppers. One alternative is the brand called Lady Poppers, available from several online shops and featuring a pink label with a ♀ symbol. The product descriptions for Lady Poppers, or any other brand for that matter, do not mention the possible use as a dysmenorrhoea relief. Perhaps manufacturers dare not follow in Routh's footsteps in caring for people with period pain for two reasons. First, the restrictive legal status of poppers, leading to the fact that the product's endurance can only really rely on word of mouth rather than the more official profile gained through advertising. Second, shame, specifically the poison of period shame. A person going to the toilet in an office usually chooses to carry their tampon or sanitary pad concealed rather than out in the open. And few people suffering period pain would excuse themselves from, say, a working day, by openly acknowledging why. Our social values and structures have far too little respect for bodies that have periods, creating shame, introducing poison.

Is period pain going to last into another century as something that people struggle with, and feel ashamed to admit to? The ultimate freedom for us has to be something like allowing ourselves to recognise the full scope of experience in having a body, the potential of our bodies, and the breadth of our desires. Being fluid, never constant, always curious. Always alternative to the ways of thinking and doing and living. The more we counteract these things that try to hold us back, the closer we come to queer utopia.

One of my poisons that really began to affect me as a teenager was the inner homophobia that I picked up somewhere or from someone. I decided to keep my wrist stiff and my knees apart, to try to pass as straight. Another: the fear of illness and death. Yet another: my own prejudice about gays. And, ultimately, another poison that afflicts me today is the very categorisation that I proudly use to assert who I am despite knowing that no legal fiction or marketable demographic can explain how it feels to be me. I agree with the women of the Combahee River Collective that emancipation requires us to think about distinct categories. We must bring everyone along on the road to freedom. But that journey is in our minds, individually and collectively. We make a mess if we try to build a certain ideal place or time.

As SOPHIE knew, every human vibrates to their own unique rhythm or, if you like, our feelings. That is why we must turn to those around us who touch queer utopia, which is really just a way of thinking honestly and deeply about ourselves, our bodies and our desires. Writers, artists and performers are particularly good at that. Queer utopia is certainly not a vision for how things should be. It is a way of disabling our poisons – right now – atom by atom.

I've borrowed my mum's Green Peugeot 206. We've parked in front of your parents' semi-detached house. It's time for you to go home. Gone midnight, and we've got college tomorrow. Yet here we are, waiting. Sometimes I think about the version of my body that touched you then. It is a version that never came to exist, a version that would have sprung out of that small car into a louche tomorrow. But I waited. I waited through my twenties, when it would have been easy to be anonymous. I waited through the coming of the apps, when I could have handpicked anyone. Every day brought an opportunity for a different version of me.

Sometimes I think about this. Sometimes I think about that decade between knowing what my body wanted in the car that night and doing what it did much later. But facing forwards is better. I don't want to dream in reverse.

9. The Next Forty-Five Seconds

There is a legend that poppers vapour was once pumped into the air over dancefloors in Manhattan. The story turns up regularly in hastily written online articles about poppers, and even in a few books. It is linked to several nightclubs, most famously with Studio 54. This place was the hot ticket in town for a few years, starting in the late 1970s, before its owners were jailed for tax evasion. The story fits with ideas of New York and Studio 54 as sinkholes for coolness and excess. Everyone who made it into that club was desirable, or at least rich and famous. Everyone was ready to focus on their pleasure. Glamour, wealth, fame, drugs... Everything was possible. They were the alien-gendered Grace Jones and David Bowie. If there truly was poppers vapour in the air, it was just there as fuel to propel them into a cosmic future a little bit faster.

That scene is all in the past, but this idea of pumping pleasure into a nightclub sticks with us like a meme. It is the basis for a section in a film called *The Fathers Project*, made by Leo Herrera and released in 2020. Herrera's film imagines a future for poppers like the probably-true one from Studio 54, but with added sexual freedom. *The Fathers Project* presents an alternative future in which HIV had never existed. Millions of lives were spared, and sex was never hampered by the virus. Artists such as Robert Mapplethorpe and Keith Haring lived on, producing more work that challenged us to think in surprising ways about our bodies. LGBTQ+ people founded an autonomous network of "Stonewall Nations" in places like Oregon and

New York, while also exercising power over federal politics. A gay president was elected...

Among all these fun imaginaries, it's Herrera's use of poppers that reveals the most about how he thinks about the past and the future. Those small poppers bottles seem to contain the potential to travel freely through thoughts and bodies. Poppers have such a power over gay culture and gay imaginations. Following this tradition, Herrera invents a future use of poppers that is based on the Studio 54 story from the past and his hope for a future life without disease.

In the film, which is fictional but takes the form of a documentary, poppers become a huge part of the mainstream club scene through the 1990s. They do not stay confined to gay sub-culture, as is largely the case in the real world we know. The brand Rush is even advertised on daytime television. But by the end of the 1990s, in this alternative timeline, sexually transmitted infections pose a real threat, as HIV can in our real world. So the Stonewall Nations fund the development of a prophylactic medicine that protects against all STIs with just a sniff. It is hailed in the film as "the most innovative medical advancement since antibiotics". Herrera branded it Espera, a name that contains multiple futures as it derives from Spanish words pertaining to waiting, hoping, or expecting.

The health authorities of the Stonewall Nations buy up Espera because the pharmaceutical manufacturer of the drug charges more for it than most individuals can afford. The nations' socialised healthcare is described in the film as "radical". To paraphrase the critic Fredric Jameson, it is easier to imagine the end of venereal disease than the end of capitalism. *The Fathers Project* contains a fake pharmaceutical ad, in the style you see on television in the USA. It features stock images of healthy, smiling, mostly white people being successful at riding up escalators and

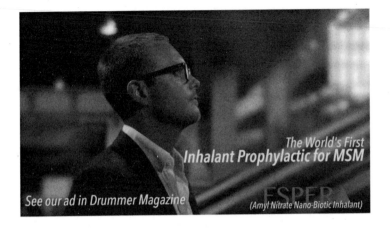

The World's First
Inhalant Prophylactic for MSM

See our ad in Drummer Magazine

ESPER

(Amyl Nitrate Nano-Biotic Inhalant)

looking at the sun. "Talk to your health provider, and discover if Espera is a fit for you," says the calming voiceover.

It's fun to look at this all through Herrera's lens, and it gets even more attractive when he pans his camera around to the dancing and fucking of nightlife. In his story, a travelling circuit party called the Quarantine takes off as the main distribution method for Espera. "Throughout the evening the prophylactic was dispensed through the ventilation system of the nightclub," says the narrator, who speaks in a robot voice. The clubs are depicted as masses of men. Muscles, leather harnesses, beards, bellies – these seem to be the dominant body symbols of the future nightlife, even though they are only a narrow depiction of what, and who, is possible. There are no scenes of mixed genders and sexes, or even of a space for queer womxn, which would hardly be a future worth having. Nevertheless, without defining who exactly is shielded by Espera, the narrator says, "Thousands were protected against all sexually transmitted diseases, free of charge. For the first time in history, disease would have no dominion over sex."

What a perfect idea. HIV and the wider microfauna of bacteria, viruses and parasites, which move between people when they fuck, have too much power. They are a poison. It is a fight for survival, and thankfully humans have bigger brains and we enjoy sex more than these bugs. Herrera opens his audience's mind to the fact that the problem of these bugs is something we can solve, and should want to. Perhaps it does not seem like a problem to many people, perhaps those who live in exclusive relationships without the threat of an STI. To be one of two partners who wouldn't test positive for any sex disease is a perfect state – call it "double-negative monogamy". But for those who live their lives outside of double-negative monogamy, as many people have long done, disease and the fear of it are huge impediments. This is the idea Herrera is exploring in his imagined future. He wants to propel us all, rightly, into a time where people can decide whether to slip a cheeky finger at the back of the bus without having to calculate a health risk. What a perfect idea.

Herrera's hopes are right about disease. But *The Fathers Project* is not the best way to think about the future, because it looks only backwards. It works as a love letter to our queer elders, those who lived their bodies in ways that help us to live ours today. It is named for men like Mapplethorpe and Haring, the "fathers" of the title. And it pays tribute to those souls whose bodies were taken from them by disease. This means that the film is not really about how to live in the future as much as it is about wishing the old trajectories had continued. Herrera wanted to build queer utopia, and he managed to remove the poison of disease from it – but he made no progress on opening up the future to different bodies. There is no space in his imagined nightclubs for lots of non-binary people, women, lesbians, people with disabilities, or even skinny gay guys who swish. Herrera's film depicts a utopia for some, but it is not queer utopia. Clearly all these distinctions still matter in the Stonewall Nations if the people who they describe don't feel welcome in the nightclubs. This is a flaw in Herrera's project, and it was created when he decided to base his imagined future on past trajectories. The pose you need to strike in order to dream of Herrera's future is a backward-looking one. I'd like this chapter to be, instead, a way of thinking about the future.

Herrera's kind of imagining is typical of science-fiction. Espera definitely fits within the tradition, as a dream that could come true. Some people say sci-fi is stupid, but that's because they've seen too much of *Star Wars*. Really, sci-fi is an artist's glimpse of a destination where we might be going to, for good or bad. In Herrera's case, it's all good, and it's based on the past. He takes a piece of history and converts it into fiction so some of us might imagine a better future. That's a decent project, and a staple of sci-fi. Rita Indiana's novel *Tentacle* does this really well too. It is set in the future, but when the protagonist takes an injection that causes an instantaneous sex change, they discover they also travel back and forth in time in order to save the coral reefs. The difference between *The Fathers Project* and *Tentacle* is that the latter is not at all nostalgic. This has to be a better footing from which to leap into tomorrow.

These stories are all about creating a future, first through imagining how we could live. We might set the bar as high as this: how we can find a way to embody queer utopia, by working to remove our poisons one by one? Disease should be first, as it is the easiest. Scientists are working on it. Hardest is next: our attitudes and the way we view each other. Performance art, like *16.97056274847714* by Luis Amália from Chapter 1, is especially good at doing this with regard to our bodies. Amália was a gymnast and an actress with a non-binary hairy body perceived as male, performing on a line among a crowd of unwitting strangers. Watching the performance, or just trying to avoid it, each viewer glimpsed an alternative way to use their own body outside any categorisation. As Amália showed, the future we want to see can be created now, imagined by our artists. The author Ray Bradbury thought the same. He wrote of the future in "The Toynbee Convector", his short story from 1984, that "what seems a lie is a ramshackle need, wishing to be born".[1]

Bradbury's story does not contain poppers, but you might imagine that the fictional society it portrays would; the things they do have include clean lakes and rivers, colonies on Mars, smog-free air, a cure for cancer, beautiful cities, and lots of whales. But all this is built on a lie, and that idea has gone on to inspire countless sci-fi writers including Iain M. Banks, author of the Culture novels. "The Toynbee Convector" centres around a 130-year-old man called Craig Bennett Stiles. One hundred years ago, Stiles created a time machine and visited the future. Upon his return he showed his fellow citizens evidence that the future contains marvellous technologies, vibrant societies and a healthy natural environment. They could not dispute his claims, which inspired them so much that they set about the enterprise of reaching the better time visited by Stiles. After a century, the time traveller reveals to a journalist that he made the whole thing up.

"You see the point, don't you, son?" Stiles asks the dumbstruck reporter. "Life has always been lying to ourselves! As boys, young men, old men. As girls, maidens, women, to gently lie and prove the lie true. To weave dreams and put brains and ideas and flesh and the truly real beneath the dreams. Everything, finally, is a promise."

With this line, Bradbury adds a twist to his own utopia but also codifies a practice of sci-fi writers. Gene Roddenberry had been up to the same thing eighteen years before Bradbury's story, when he created *Star Trek* in 1966. The human corners of the universes in *Star Trek* and "The Toynbee Convector" are desirable – healthy people in ordered societies. (In *Star Trek*, other species are not so well balanced, hence the drama.) The world of *The Fathers Project* sits in the same orbit as Bradbury's and Roddenberry's. It is a promise of a better future – a lie, yes, but one that will become true if we can only imagine it, and include all bodies in our scope. This chapter itself is an exercise in doing the same. It is not a prediction of *the* future; it is a way of imagining *a* future.

The story of poppers is filled with dreams about the future. And if we hunt through the past, we can find the presence of poppers vapour in the most significant developments of the industrial world. At first, the substance was a useless poison in the early nineteenth century when scientists were discovering many such things. But as science and medicine joined up, and medicine itself codified into evidence-based therapies, Thomas Lauder Brunton picked up amyl nitrite and made it mean something. It relieved the suffering of his angina patients, and he used medical journals in the late nineteenth century to popularise his therapy. This practice of discovery-and-dissemination remains a pillar of science and technology. It is an astonishingly successful method at removing poisons like disease.

The technologies of manufacturing and distribution created a viable and cost-effective pharmaceutical product out of amyl nitrite, and brought it into the twentieth century. That is the story of commercialisation, through investment, marketing, sales – thanks to capitalism. The proliferation of this product raised a sub-culture of alternative uses, largely gay men looking to open their bumholes and feel a head rush. As sexual freedoms through the 1950s, 60s and 70s expanded, so did use of poppers. Even when sex was halted for gay men in the 80s, poppers were present. Indeed, poppers were believed to be the obstacle, the cause of the awful affliction known first as AIDS. Now they are back – on our dancefloors, in our sex shops and in our porn.

Although poppers are heavily associated with gay men, as *The Fathers Project* shows, new sub-cultures are using them in new ways, offering a fascinating glimpse at their longevity and their future.

This all sounds mad. Poppers? At the heart of all these developments in rich, Western society? Really? Poppers may not have driven any of these trends, but they were present. They endure because of the feeling they give. Plenty of products with better reputations and broader marketing have failed simply because they were not good enough. But the vapour of poppers is still among us, and will remain so, because it works.

So, where next for poppers? How do we think about a future? We must return to *Star Trek* – not because it presents a viable or even desirable vision, but because in the future we are all shapeshifters.

One of the most fascinating characters in more than fifty years and countless hours of *Star Trek* is Odo, whose body can take any form. Odo featured in the *Deep Space Nine* television series from 1993 to 1999 and was portrayed as male, even though members of Odo's species don't have penises, vaginas or a concept of gender. If *Deep Space Nine* were remade today, the producers would hopefully portray the character as neither male nor female, or both, or non-binary, with the pronouns they/them. Perhaps Odo would not use pronouns at all, like SOPHIE. In the 1990s, *Star Trek* did not even portray homosexuality without heavy coding, so Odo was forced to take the form of a man and when "he" eventually came to desire others, they were only female "solid" people. Today it is close to the queer spirit of Odo to see them without the boundaries of human sex and gender, and to use them/they pronouns when writing about them. In 2020, a non-binary human character named Adira Tal joined the most recent series, *Star Trek: Discovery*. Their body hosts a symbiotic life-form that carries the memories of the deceased men and women who were its previous hosts.

Backstory is important to Odo, too, and they certainly have a lot of it before the events on *Deep Space Nine* began. Odo is from a species which does not usually live as separate individuals, but as a gelatinous oceanic mass the colour of bronze. It is known as The Great Link, and it means that the entire species experiences the same things at the same time. Due to the constraints of easy-watching evening television, parts of the species separate off and take the form of an individual like Odo, played by a human actor in a latex mask. Such individuals in the show are known as Changelings. I use they/them pronouns for Odo not only to reflect the genderqueer nature of their species, but also as a way of referring to the fact that their species usually lives communally, as a plural.

Odo is different, living as an individual after having been severed from The Great Link and sent off into space years ago. Found by a scientist, Odo endured experiments until they formed a part of their body into a tentacle and batted off the captor. Lost from their home planet, Odo lives as an isolated Changeling in a galaxy of solid people. They live as a pretend solid person too, every day forming a body shape like a human's and every night returning to a gelatinous state in a bucket. That is pretty weird, and not the only reason why Changelings have a bad reputation. Their species is known for vicious tyranny on account of having created servile soldier races with which to dominate the galaxy. This means that even though Odo is separated from their people, they face prejudice and suspicion among "solids". They are vilified when they just want to be accepted. They are full of potential as they are constrained by solids. Like poppers, they are able to live as liquid and vapour.

Odo is one of the queerest characters in popular culture simply because of how different they are from everyone else around. Odo embodies the idea of being queer as a feeling, an experience and a relative position – nothing to do with a solid category. One way the show's writers portray Odo as different from solids in the earlier episodes of the series is their lack of sexual drive, usually played for comedy. "I have no desire to become a slave to humanoid obsessions," Odo says in "Broken Link" in season four.

By season seven, Odo is fully accepted among the main group of characters and is even in a relationship with a solid woman called Kira. Odo has earned respect as a law enforcer and an asset in a war against the bad guys. But they are shocked when another Changeling, Laas, arrives in the episode "Chimera" and tells the truth about Odo's adoptive society. "They tolerate you, Odo," says Laas, "because you emulate them... they know that you are truly not one of them."

Laas proposes to Odo that together they form a new Great Link, but the producers of *Deep Space Nine* must have been too coy. They skipped over the chance to create the first non-solid gender-neutral-multi-sex couple on television. Joined, Laas and Odo would have sought other Changelings to merge into their new Great Link. Even though Odo's species are actually waging a war, which I'm not going to go into here, theoretically their nature means they can live plurally, communally, in queer utopia. I want to believe that this is in our nature too. But *Deep Space Nine* was just a US television show, so Odo finds a solid woman to pair off with. The episode ends with Odo and Kira having a kind of sex, although there is no word in the show for what they do. Odo's body turns into something that is both light and vapour, a sexy glowing steam that envelops Kira. She twirls and grins like a woman in an advert for Herbal Essences shampoo. She seems to have the same sensual-sexual experience in the presence of vapour as the patrons of Studio 54 might have done in the late 1970s.

Much of Odo's arc over seven seasons is a search for identity – that is, their homeland and their people. But "their people" turn out to be an oozing bronze gelatinous mass that started a war to enslave the galaxy. Plus Odo is an individual, and one with the ethics to know that imperialism is wrong. So what is Odo's identity really? Much of it actually comes from their survival of trauma and rejection, their coping as an outsider, their strong sense of justice, and their job in law enforcement. Odo's idea of homeland and of 'their' people are really just categories. These ideas don't fit with the feeling of *being* Odo.

Really Odo's quest is not about finding a "true" identity. It is about reaching the level of self-respect they need in order to be comfortable in their natural state. Odo's natural state is literally fluid. When Laas wants him and Odo to make themselves fluid so they can 'link' on the public promenade of the space station, Odo refuses: "I don't want to do something that might make people uncomfortable." By the end of that episode, in private, Odo finds a way of being naturally a Changeling but with another person, when they turn into vapour and give Kira a sexy steam bath. Being comfortable with another person means flowing on and around her, as Odo does with Kira. In this moment, Odo's customary humanoid form means nothing because it is not truly Odo anyway. Their supposed identity as a member of a liquid species means nothing because they are capable of alternative connection. It is all intensely metaphorical, never more so than when Odo gives Kira pleasure through the medium of vapour.

On the actual Earth, in the actual twentieth century, gay men were vilified as being unnatural in nature, a threat to physical safety and social harmony. Ditto other people in the QUILTBAG. From the moment that people of difference are categorised, others find it easier to say that those people don't belong. Odo doesn't belong either, even though they live in the twenty-fourth century. Odo is rejected for the same reasons that QUILTBAG people on Earth have been.

Chapter 2 explored how gay men were excluded from mainstream society in countries with a classically liberal tradition, and their response to conceive of themselves as individuals with an immutable identity. Identity is present in such men by their nature as homosexual – this is an argument made by Karl Heinrich Ulrichs in his talks and pamplets in Germany from around 1867 and later. On top of this came the political arguments about a group identity, formed through a shared oppression, culture and consumerism. By the 1970s, gay men were being persuaded by advertising that poppers were an integral part of their identity. Adverts showed idealised and sexualised male bodies, and wishful concepts of power and strength. You are what you buy. Nothing could be gayer and manlier than huffing fumes in an endurance trial. "Looking for muscular or fit submissive/horny popperfaggot who wants to be coached," says a user on popperbate.com.

Today, poppers ads seem to display offer codes more frequently than they do bodies, but they keep a firm place within capitalism among plenty of products marketed specifically at people in the category of "gay men". Kinky harnesses for buff bodies. A rainbow Christmas tree bauble personalised with the names and skin tones of two gay husbands. The "essential viewing" of the latest algorithmically written gay drama on Netflix. Life insurance for married gays ("protect your partner for just 20p a day"). But categories and demographics are so limiting. As Odo knows, no one truly fits. Signifiers never really match what they signify – would the partner covered by the life insurance ever really feel *protected*?

Somehow identities are a part of capitalism, subject to marketing, as those early poppers adverts pioneered. But the thing about poppers, like most drugs, is that they also help people to escape this truth briefly. Drew Gregory, a filmmaker, describes this unique pleasure:

> I want to live in a world where I'm not the only trans woman in dykey spaces or the only dyke in faggoty spaces. I want to live in a world where the terms AFAB [assigned female at birth] and AMAB [assigned male at birth] are obsolete. I want to live in a world that feels as queer as I do. I want to live in a world without dysphoria. I want to live in that moment I inhale chemicals out of a bottle. I want to live in those forty-five seconds when it all feels possible.[2]

Gregory implies that there is nothing gay about sniffing poppers. There is really only a feeling, not an identity at all. But a feeling needs to be somewhat solid in order to be talked about and understood. That is why Ulrichs declared his *identity* as a man who desires other men – to make it possible to express this as a legal *category* in order for certain humans to have their rights respected. Ulrichs' friend Karl-Maria Kertbeny did the work here, codifying his and Ulrichs' feeling of who they were into the word "homosexual". He therefore created the "heterosexual" too, and boundaries were drawn. We can thank the two Karls for what they were trying to do. But the fact is that the categories they created, and the ones the great marketers of the twentieth century worked with, are now creaking.

Respecting different identities within a society and even within an individual is both a solution and a problem. It is a solution because it allows people a chance to live freely. And it is a problem because dividing people into categories – the things that products can be sold to – feels like a way to distance ourselves from ourselves, from the "possible" future that Gregory seeks, a future without boundaries. We are, in fact, full of surprises. You only have to look at two examples from the characters in this book to know that.

Pete Fisher agitated for gay pleasure in 1970s New York as an activist and included poppers in *Dreamlovers*, a fictional depiction of the era mentioned in Chapters 1 and 3. At some point Fisher turned his brain to *Star Trek* fan fiction. In 1977, he wrote an unofficial novel called *Black Star* in which a male trucker from Earth gets beamed aboard the *USS Enterprise* for a fling with Captain Kirk, even though non-reproductive sex is *verboten*.[3] "How do you think we keep ourselves entertained on those long treks through space?" says comms officer Uhura. "Basket weaving? People keep fairly quiet about it... for a lot of reasons."

And Brunton, the doctor who developed a treatment for angina with amyl nitrite, has yet another surprise. Brunton was raised as a Christian in Scotland, trained as a medical doctor and made an English Baronet in 1909. In his later years he became a Muslim and changed his name to Jalaluddin. "I pondered over the matter a great deal," he wrote in his contribution to a pamphlet about converts entitled *Islam – Our Choice*, published by the Muslim World League.[4] Brunton explained his distaste for Christians' vilification of the prophet Muhammad, who, he learnt, had furnished his followers with dignity and cleanliness. "[I] brought one argument after the other bearing upon the Christians' present day religion and I concluded in favour of Islam, feeling convinced of its truth, simplicity, toleration, sincerity and brotherhood."

The lives of Brunton and Fisher, and many more in these pages, exhibit the flexibility of the human. Something about the way we live means that we trap our soul and our nature into categories. This is not the future we deserve. If I feel like a "man" who is "gay", I have to wonder about the solidity of those words, and therefore their usefulness. Better to be fluid, like Odo. "What drew (and draws) me to science fiction is simple: bending," wrote So Mayer in an essay called *Space Orchids* in 2020.[5] I stand, and mince and flow, with Mayer, inhabiting the "bending time, bending bodies".

But on dating apps, the homosexuals conceived by Kertbeny and Ulrichs have become another product for sale: a top, a bottom, a racialised fantasy, a piggy sub fag... Heterosexuals don't seem to share this need to divide themselves further and further, but gay men seem to have been destined for it ever since the innovations of Kertbeny and Ulrichs. Today any manifestation of a person's queerness is bunched with that of and compared to others'. This is how a queer soul can still feel left aside by 'queer culture'. Somehow our souls do not fit into the human boxes we make, so we try to make our souls solid, with products, films, phrases. Really we're looking for a release from all of that, a connection beyond. Between bators who meet in virtual rooms to wank and huff together, there is a connection that travels via electrons and cables and network routers. But the thing that makes those meetings so necessary to bators is the actual physical and emotional feelings they experience in their own bodies, on their own side of the screen, the subjective sensation of sex.

Poppers are both a product and the thing we use to release our souls. Like any drug, poppers help us to believe we've escaped our material circumstances. That escape is only ever brief, like the relief from angina or period pain. For gay men or some queer people, poppers carry the added benefit of a shared history, part of a culture, a group experience. Sniffing can also feel extreme for those who want that, with trainer videos and masks that force deep inhalation. People who want to open their bumholes can achieve that too. We inhale from our little bottles because we just want to be free of our bodies. We know deep down a truth about our bodies: they are the material that gives other people a hundred reasons to categorise us. Really we want to be vapour, like Odo in their most transcendental moment. We want the world to see the real us. You might call this our soul.

A better future is like a poppered-up body's bumhole: open. The future is best when it is open to surprise and connection, not based on a thing that didn't happen in the past, as in *The Fathers Project*. Nor is the future a bunch of different sentient species strolling around a space station, even though the diversity of bodies offered in that image is something for us to plan. Instead, the future is a feeling inside each of us, a dream, a desire, a promise to be ourselves. The future is who we become in the next forty-five seconds. Us mortal humans can only try to get to the queer utopia that Odo and Amália actually seemed to embody.

You came for a history, but I'd rather you leave with a future. I do not mean only concrete things like rights and possessions. Or fantasies like living in space. I mean a future of feeling. Poppers gives the sensation of connection and of possibility. Gregory is right to chase the forty-five seconds. Let's live there. It's so close but full of potential. Humans can push towards that queer future, where alternative voices are heard and respected, new pleasures discovered, surprising connections made. Meet me in the next forty-five seconds.

References

Sections of the work in this book that draw directly from others' work are referenced in these endnotes. The titles that informed this work generally are listed in the Books section that follows.

Endnotes

1. Undesirable Purposes

1 https://vimeo.com/428267625
2 *The Chemist and Druggist*, July 29th, 1978
3 *The Chemist and Druggist*, July 31st, 1976
4 *The Chemist and Druggist*, July 29th, 1978
5 Switchboard log book archive, held in the Bishopsgate Institute, ref: Nov-Mar 1975-6, SB/5/1/3
6 Switchboard log book archive, held in the Bishopsgate Institute, ref: Mar-Jul 1976, SB/5/1/4
7 Today the book is titled *Martindale: The Complete Drug Reference*, and it is updated and re-published by Pharmaceutical Press every two years.
8 Today the book is titled *Martindale: The Complete Drug Reference*, and it is updated and re-published by Pharmaceutical Press every two years.
9 *The Chemist and Druggist*, December 29th, 1956
10 Sansweet, Stephen J., "A New Way to Glow and Giggle, and Get A Headache Besides", *Wall Street Journal*, October 10th, 1977, https://bit.ly/3eihtjw
11 Fritscher, Jack, *Gay Pioneers: How Drummer Magazine Shaped Gay Popular Culture 1965-1999*, Palm Drive Publishing, 2017

12 Fritscher, Jack, *Gay Pioneers: How Drummer Magazine Shaped Gay Popular Culture 1965-1999*, Palm Drive Publishing, 2017

13 Nickerson, Mark, et al, *ISOBUTYL NITRITE and Related Compounds*, 1979

14 Fisher, Pete, *Dreamlovers*, Sea Horse Press, 1980

15 Nickerson, Mark, et al, *ISOBUTYL NITRITE and Related Compounds*, 1979

16 White, Jane See, *Desert Sun*, "'Disco drug' dangers debated", September 17, 1979, https://bit.ly/3gEYmmD

17 *The Sentinel*, December 10th, 1981, available here: https://bit.ly/3tCLP6P

18 *Bay Area Reporter*, "Poppers Maker Dies of AIDS", May 16th, 1985, https://bit.ly/32LTUdD

19 Consumer Product Safety Commission, "Great Lakes Products Inc. Pays to Settle Civil Penalty Case", September 22nd, 1994

20 Preciado, Paul B, *Testo Junkie*, Feminist Press at the City University of New York, 2019 (originally published as *Testo Yonqui* in 2008 by Espasa Calpe in Madrid)

21 UK government, "Drug Misuse: Findings from the 2015/16 Crime Survey for England and Wales", July 2016: https://bit.ly/32ygrdz

22 Scott, Richard, "Oh my Soho", from *Soho*, Faber, 2018

2. Two Body Innovators

1 Dormandy, Thomas, *The Worst of Evils: The Fight Against Pain,* Yale University Press, 2006

2 Brunton, Thomas Lauder, "On the use of nitrite of amyl in angina pectoris", *The Lancet*, July 27th, 1867

3 Fye, W.B., "Profiles in Cardiology: T. Lauder Brunton, 1844-1916", in *Clinical Cardiology*, 1989

4 Brunton, Thomas Lauder, "Nitrite of Amyl in Angina

Pectoris", *Journal of Anatomy and Physiology*, Vol V, Feb 1870, reprinted from the *Clinical Society's Reports*, Vol III

5   Beachy, Robert, *Gay Berlin*, Vintage, 2014
6   *The Chemist and Druggist*, September 23rd, 1916
7   *The Chemist and Druggist*, December 15th, 1888
8   Fye, W.B., "T. Lauder Brunton and amyl nitrite: a Victorian vasodilator", in *Circulation*, August 1986
9   Muñoz, José Esteban, *Cruising Utopia*, New York University Press, 2009

3. The Creation of Man?

1   http://www.fonda.org/index.htm
2   *British Medical Journal*, "Poisoning by Amyl-Nitrite", November 27th, 1880, available here: https://bit.ly/2QMtipN
3   *Bronxville Review Press and Reporter*, "Howard B. Fonda, Retired Executive, Dies At Age 68", March 12th, 1964, https://bit.ly/2RVtXWR
4   Young, Ian, *The Stonewall Experiment*, Cassell, 1995
5   Young, Ian, *The Stonewall Experiment*, Cassell, 1995
6   Israelstam, Stephen, Lambert, Sylvia, and Oki, Gustav, "Poppers, a new recreational drug craze", *Canadian Psychiatric Association Journal*, 1978
7   Fritscher, Jack, Gay Pioneers: How Drummer Magazine Shaped Gay Popular Culture 1965-1999, Palm Drive Publishing, 2017
8   Young, Ian, *The Stonewall Experiment*, Cassell, 1995
9   *Heaven (Gay Life)*, made by London Weekend Television, 1980, https://bit.ly/2QjUa0G

4. Sex / Death

1   Haverkos (ed.), Health Hazards on Nitrite Inhalants, Research Series Monograph, National Institute on Drug Abuse 1988

2   Switchboard log book archive, held in the Bishopsgate Institute, ref: Aug-Nov 1975, SB/5/1/2

3   Switchboard log book archive, held in the Bishopsgate Institute, ref: Aug-Nov 1975, SB/5/1/2

4   Durack, David T., *New England Journal of Medicine*, December 10th, 1981

5   McManus, T.J., "Letter: similar use incidence in UK as in US", *The Lancet*, 1982

6   *Killer in the Village*, BBC, first broadcast on April 25th, 1983, https://bbc.in/2QNfMm8

7   *The Log Books* podcast, season 2, episode 1

8   Berg, P., "Use of 'Poppers' Linked to Kaposi's Sarcoma", *Washington Post*, April 24th, 1985

9   Lauritsen, J. and Wilson H., *Death Rush: Poppers and AIDS*, Pagan Press, New York, 1986

10 Anti-Drug Abuse Act of 1988, https://bit.ly/3tGD0IU

11 *Capital Gay*, April 7th, 1989

12 Crime Control Act of 1990, https://bit.ly/3sBiMPD

13 *AIDS: A Strange and Deadly Virus,* BBC, 1986

14 *Capital Gay*, January 29th, 1988

15 Hansard, December 18th, 1986, https://bit.ly/3grejwp

16 Scarce, Michael, *Smearing the Queer*, Haworth Press, 1999

17 Rewbury R., Hughes E., Purbrick R., "Poppers: legal highs with questionable contents? A case series of poppers maculopathy", *British Journal of Ophthalmology*, May 2017

5. Utopia for a Moment

1   GALOP annual report, 1986-87, https://bit.ly/3n84SDt

2   *Associated Press*, "3 Jailed in Cases Linked to Overdose Death of Cabinet Minister's Daughter", December 5th, 1986, https://bit.ly/3gxSmfn

3   *The Log Books* podcast, season 2, episode 6
4   Walters, Ben, "The police wore rubber gloves", January 17th, 2017, available here: https://bit.ly/3vdDWoN
5   *Capital Gay*, January 9th, 1987
6   Burston, Paul, "*Time Out* Tells the Remarkable Story of a True London Survivor", *Time Out*, January 2007, https://bit.ly/3xnhR98
7   SB Log book, Dec-Feb 1986-7, SB/5/1/25
8   *Heart of the Matter*, BBC, March 8th, 1987
9   *Capital Gay*, April 1st, 1988 and Aug 26th, 1988
10 Silversides, Ann, *AIDS Activist*, Between the Lines, 2003
11 Hansard, February 2nd, 1987, https://bit.ly/3eCNUqQ
12 *Capital Gay*, February 6th, 1987
13 *The Independent* obituaries, October 23rd, 2011, https://bit.ly/3sH4Gfn
14 Hansard, December 18th, 1986, https://bit.ly/3v7cJ78
15 *Gay Rights – The London Programme*, LWT, October 4th, 1987
16 *Capital Gay*, April 24th, 1987
17 *Capital Gay*, December 18th, 1987
18 *Capital Gay*, June 10th, 1988
19 *Capital Gay*, March 17th, 1989
20 Works by Jade Pollard-Crowe, https://bit.ly/2P6Gs0r

6. A Guilty Pleasure

1   Dan Goggin on the creation of *Nunsense*, Concord Theatricals, July 28th, 2015, https://bit.ly/3ei2OEQ
2   *Sun*, March 6th, 1989
3   *Daily Mail*, "Gordon Ramsay's 'seven-year affair': TV chef who fostered a family image is accused of adultery", November 24th, 2008, https://bit.ly/3sCsFfU
4   Milton, Josh, "Ally of the year Nicole Scherzinger 'sniffed poppers' at a gay bar with Sam Smith and we

have no legal choice but to stan", *PinkNews*, December 14th, 2019, https://bit.ly/3tFoT6J

5 Padgett, Donald, "Sam Smith Finally Addresses Rumors About Doing Poppers in a Club", *Out.com*, April 22nd, 2020, https://bit.ly/3n8addL

6 Fagen, Cynthia R., "JFK's teen mistress addresses relationship in memoir", *New York Post*, February 5th, 2012, https://bit.ly/2RQvQUC

7 Coleman, Oli, "New interview sheds light on the life of the late Brigid Berlin", *Page Six*, July 25th, 2020, https://pge.sx/3v8hq0e

8 Doyle, Arthur Conan, *The Resident Patient*, originally published in *The Strand Magazine*, 1893

9 *Mes Chéris*, directed by Ethan Folk and Ty Wardwell, Cutenon Films, 2020

10 *Lemon Taste*, directed by Nicky Miller, 2018

11 Hansard, January 20th, 2016, https://bit.ly/2QJWjTj

12 Liddle, Rod, "Did we really have to hear all about Crispin Blunt's sex life?", *Spectator* blog, January 25th, 2016, https://bit.ly/3vc7HGv

7. HIT / HOLD / RELEASE

1 Townsend, Larry, *The Leatherman's Handbook*, LT Publications, 1972

2 Townsend, Larry, *Leatherman's Workbook 5*, LT Publications, 1976

3 Delany, Samuel R, *Times Square Red, Times Square Blue*, New York University Press, 1999

8. Antidote

1 Gay Liberation Front Manifesto, 1971 (UK)

2 Mitchell, Larry and Ned Asta, *The Faggots and Their Friends Between Revolutions*, Nightboat Books, 2019, first published by Calamus Books in 1977

3 https://bit.ly/3dzGdo0

4   https://bit.ly/32ArTW0

5   *The Chemist and Druggist*, December 29th, 1956

6   Cataldie, Louis, letter to the *Journal of the American Medical Association*, May

7   https://bit.ly/2PdAOtG

8   Today the book is titled *Martindale: The Complete Drug Reference*, and it is updated and re-published by Pharmaceutical Press every two years.

9   Routh, Amand, "A Lecture on Dysmenorrhoea", *British Medical Journal*, August 4th, 1906

9. The Next Forty-Five Seconds

1   Bradbury, Ray, "The Toynbee Convector", first published in *Playboy* magazine in 1984

2   Gregory, Drew, "Giving Poppers to Cis Women", *Autostraddle*, October 19th, 2020, https://bit.ly/3sL8ZGV

3   Fisher, Pete, *Black Star*, published by Unrepressed Press and Shoestring Press in 1983

4   *Islam - Our Choice: Impressions of Eminent Converts to Islam*, compiled and edited by Ebrahim Ahmed Bawany, no date, https://bit.ly/2PdAH1e. Brunton's conversion is also mentioned by Angus Mitchell in his history of Brunton's wife's family, *The Stopfords of Blackwater House: Alice Stopford Green's Family Circle*, 2019, https://bit.ly/3sDKVph

5   Mayer, So, *Space Orchids* in *In the Past the Future Was Better*, published by Cipher Press, 2020

Books

Histories
Gay Bar: Why We Went Out by Jeremy Atherton Lin, Granta, 2021

Gay Berlin by Robert Beachy, Vintage, 2014

Stand by Me by Jim Downs, Basic Books, 2016

Cruising by Alex Espinoza, Unnamed Press, 2019

Gay Pioneers: How Drummer Magazine Shaped Gay Popular Culture 1965-1999 by Jack Fritscher, Palm Drive Publishing, 2017

Buying Gay: How Physique Entrepreneurs Sparked a Movement by David K. Johnson, Columbia University Press, 2019

AIDS Activist by Ann Silversides, Between the Lines, 2003

Policing Desire by Simon Watney, Methuen & Co, 1987

The Stonewall Experiment by Ian Young, Cassell, 1995

Stories
Matter by Iain M. Banks, Orbit, 2008

The Hours by Michael Cunningham, Farrar, Straus and Giroux, 1998

Cleanness by Garth Greenwell, Picador, 2020

Tentacle by Rita Indiana, And Other Stories, 2018

Dance: Ten Murder: Maybe? by Ken Landsdowne, 2012

Box Hill by Adam Mars-Jones, Fitzcarraldo Editions, 2020

The Argonauts by Maggie Nelson, Melville House, 2015

Soho by Richard Scott, Faber, 2018

Revolutionary Road by Richard Yates, Little, Brown and Company, 1961

Ideas
What's the Use? by Sara Ahmed, Duke University Press, 2019

Go the Way Your Blood Beats by Michael Amherst, Repeater Books, 2018

Times Square Red, Times Square Blue by Samuel R. Delany, New York University Press, 1999

No Future by Lee Edelman, Duke University Press, 2004

How to Be Gay by David Halperin, the Belknap Press of Harvard University Press, 2012

A Nazi Word for a Nazi Thing by So Mayer, Peninsula Press, 2020

Cruising Utopia by José Esteban Muñoz, New York University Press, 2009

An Apartment on Uranus by Paul B. Preciado, Fitzcarraldo Editions, 2020

Testo Junkie by Paul B. Preciado, Feminist Press at the City University of New York, 2019 (originally published as *Testo Yonqui* in 2008 by Espasa Calpe in Madrid)

Smearing the Queer: Medical Bias in the Health Care of Gay Men by Michael Scarce, Haworth Press Inc, 1999

Illness as Metaphor / AIDS and its Metaphors by Susan Sontag, 1978, 1989

The Trouble with Normal by Michael Warner

Images

1. Undesirable Purposes
- p. 2. Still from *16.97056274847714* by Luis Amália (still credit: Luis Amália)
- p. 5. Pearls of amyl nitrite (credit: Science Museum, London)

2. Two Body Innovators
- p. 22. Thomas Lauder Brunton, photograph by G. Jerrard, 1881
- p. 32. Karl Heinrich Ulrichs

3. The Creation of Man?
- p. 44. Patent - amyl nitrite inhaler
- p. 52. Bolt poppers ad, 1970s, artwork by Rex

4. Sex / Death
- p. 61. Hard Ware poppers ad from *Drummer* magazine, 1982

6. A Guilty Pleasure
- p. 103. Poppers panels by Jerry Mills, originally published in *Touch Magazine* in the 1980s

7. HIT / HOLD / RELEASE
- p. 122. Still from popperbator video by marcutureno

9. The Next Forty-Five Seconds
- p. 165. Still from *The Fathers Project*, 2020, dir Leo Herrera

Playlist

3, 2, 1... HIT.

Some of the songs mentioned in this book, and many more that are connected to poppers one way or another, feature in a playlist that is available on Spotify and Apple Music:

Spotify

Apple Music

Acknowledgements

This book has mushroomed from a talk I gave at Fringe! Queer Film & Arts Fest in November 2019. I'll be forever grateful to the unstoppable Fringe! collective for making that talk happen, and especially to Muffin Hix and the Duchess of Pork aka Alex Karotsch for letting me run with the idea in the first place. Paul Gorczynski offered thoughtful notes on the first draft of that talk, which also began to steer the ideas into what became this book.

Joel Love and Luis Amália read the chapters as they came, offering criticism, ideas and inspiration. They were essential cheerleaders of the project throughout the long writing process.

I worked with Tash Walker and Shivani Dave on *The Log Books* podcast while writing this; our research findings and conversations about queer history fed many of the ideas on these pages. Also, Tash read the manuscript and got excited about it.

Frances Lubbe and Amy Spiller offered sharp and empathetic analyses of the manuscript. They also listened to me, encouraged me and taught me things over every coffee break we had at home as I wrote it.

Peter Scalpello read an early draft of Chapter 7 and convinced me that it had something to say.

I'm in debt to the many brilliant writers whose works are named in the book list. But also to Hugh Ryan and Steven Thrasher, who both model for me how to combine the work of writing with the work of being human.

I'm grateful to the artist Bobby Redmond, who produced the extraordinarily heady poppers bottle cover art. His work is a vibrant performance of queer utopia. There are other artists, performers and makers who appear in these pages, and I thank them all.

Thank you to everyone at Repeater for making this book happen, and especially to Ellie Potts for the careful editing. Marcus Gilroy-Ware helped me to form ideas into a book proposal, while showing me how to follow through, in his own titles published by Repeater.

Shout out to Spread the Word for being a powerhouse of support for writers, including me.

For help with archival research, I want to thank: Stef Dickers and team at the Bishopsgate Institute, Switchboard – the LGBT+ Helpline, the Wellcome Library, Siân Cook, Leif Anderson at Stanford University, and Jack Fritscher who arrived with Hard Ware in the nick of time.

REPEATER BOOKS

is dedicated to the creation of a new reality. The landscape of twenty-first-century arts and letters is faded and inert, riven by fashionable cynicism, egotistical self-reference and a nostalgia for the recent past. Repeater intends to add its voice to those movements that wish to enter history and assert control over its currents, gathering together scattered and isolated voices with those who have already called for an escape from Capitalist Realism. Our desire is to publish in every sphere and genre, combining vigorous dissent and a pragmatic willingness to succeed where messianic abstraction and quiescent co-option have stalled: abstention is not an option: we are alive and we don't agree